SO-BAS-880

Patient Outcomes in Maternal-Infant Nursing

Lisa E. Rowland, RN,CS, MSN, FNP
Family Nurse Practitioner
Twin Lakes Regional Health System
Leitchfield, Kentucky

Patricia Iyer, RN, MSN, CNA
President
Patricia Iyer Associates
Stockton, New Jersey

Springhouse Corporation
Springhouse, Pennsylvania

Staff

EXECUTIVE DIRECTOR, EDITORIAL
Stanley Loeb

SENIOR PUBLISHER, TRADE AND TEXTBOOKS
Minnie. B. Rose, RN, BSN, MEd

ART DIRECTOR
John Hubbard

CLINICAL EDITOR
Patricia Kardish Fischer, RN, BSN

EDITORS
Nancy Priff (senior editor), Terri Greenberg, Cynthia Jennings, Kevin Law

ASSOCIATE ACQUISITIONS EDITOR
Caroline Lemoine

COPY EDITORS
Julie Cullen, Debra Davis, Barbara Hodgson

DESIGNERS
Stephanie Peters (associate art director), Cindy Marczuk

EDITORIAL ASSISTANT
Louise Quinn

MANUFACTURING
Deborah Meiris (director), Anna Brindisi, Kate Davis, T.A. Landis

Printed in the United States of America. For more information, write Springhouse Corporation, 1111 Bethlehem Pike, P.O. Box 908, Springhouse, PA 19477-0908.

PTOUTMAT-011094

A member of the Reed Elsevier plc group

Library of Congress Cataloging-in-Publication Data

Rowland, Lisa E.
    Patient outcomes in maternal-infant nursing/Lisa E. Rowland, Patricia Iyer.
    p. cm.
    Includes bibliographical references and index.
    1. Maternity nursing. 2. Infants (Newborn)–Diseases–Nursing. 3. Outcome Assessment (Medical Care)
    I. Iyer, Patricia W. II. Title.
    [DNLM: 1. Pregnancy Complications–nursing. 2. Outcome Assessment (Health Care)–nurses' instruction. 3. Maternal-Child Nursing. 4. Infant, Newborn, Diseases–Nursing.
    WQ 240 R883p 1994]
RG951.R68 1994
610.73'67--dc20
DNLM/DLC
                          94-22564
ISBN 0-87434-700-9   CIP

Contents

ANTEPARTAL PERIOD

INTRAPARTAL PERIOD

POSTPARTAL PERIOD

INFANT

APPENDICES, SELECTED REFERENCES, AND INDEX

Acknowledgments and Dedication

The author wishes to thank the series author, Patricia Iyer, RN, MSN, CNA, for her patient guidance; the Springhouse editors; and the following reviewer for her valuable suggestions:

Sarah E. Whitaker, RN, DNSc(C)
Lecturer
University of Texas at El Paso

Dedication

This book is dedicated with love to
Zach, Brad, and Eric Rowland,
my wind, sun, and stars.

Preface

This practical care-planning guide concentrates on the specific needs of maternity patients. Divided into four sections—antepartal, intrapartal, postpartal, and infant—the book uses a standard format for each entry:

• *Definition* describes the condition or health care concern.

• *Nursing diagnosis* focuses the plan of care.

• *Desired patient outcome* reflects the nursing diagnosis and directs all nursing care.

• *Outcome measurement criteria* provide objective, measurable elements that help the nurse determine if the goal has been met or partially met—a boon to quality assurance.

• *Key interventions* direct nursing activities that are essential to meeting the outcome measurement criteria and the patient's goal.

Appendices include the complete NANDA taxonomy of nursing diagnoses and a summary of common nursing diagnoses in maternal-infant care. They are followed by selected references (a valuable guide to sources for further information) and a detailed index.

Throughout its pages, *Patient Outcomes in Maternal-Infant Nursing* emphasizes patient teaching—one of the most important nursing interventions for maternity patients. With this book as a resource, the nurse can now easily meet the informational and health-care needs of the pregnant woman, new mother, and her newborn and family.

Adolescent pregnancy

Pregnancy that occurs during the developmental stage of adolescence.

NURSING DIAGNOSIS

Anxiety related to parenthood, the effects of parenthood on relationships, and labor and delivery

DESIRED PATIENT OUTCOME

The patient will manage anxiety effectively and demonstrate problem-solving skills

Outcome measurement criteria

☐ Verbalization of specific causes of anxiety

☐ Verbalization of effective coping skills

☐ Exploration of choices about pregnancy continuation or termination

☐ Investigation of methods for coping with labor

☐ Investigation of education options for young parents

☐ Consideration of options for continuing relationships with family and peers

☐ Participation in decisions about pregnancy

☐ Expression of satisfaction with decisions

Key interventions

• Establish a rapport with the patient and encourage her to express concerns. Be alert for indications of denial.

- Help the patient identify previously successful coping techniques.

- Describe typical concerns of pregnant adolescents and determine whether the patient shares those concerns. Lead the patient into discussion by using nonthreatening communication techniques.

- Help the patient recognize her need to make decisions about the pregnancy and to plan for herself.

- Encourage the patient to explore different ways to deal with specific anxiety-producing issues, such as telling her parents and partner about the pregnancy, managing the pregnancy, dealing with peers, dealing with body image concerns, and coping with labor.

- Help the patient review her options and make decisions about her concerns. Reinforce that she is responsible for her decisions.

- Reassess the patient's feelings about anxiety-producing issues and help her make decisions that satisfy her.

NURSING DIAGNOSIS

Altered family processes related to the stress of adolescent pregnancy

DESIRED PATIENT OUTCOME

The patient's family will manage stress effectively and develop appropriate coping mechanisms

Outcome measurement criteria

☐ Verbalization of the effect of the adolescent's pregnancy on the family

☐ Participation in problem solving related to pregnancy management

☐ Demonstration of support for the pregnant adolescent

Key interventions

- Encourage open communication among family members and health care team members. Provide a private, supportive environment for discussions.
- Help the family explore the effects of decisions related to the adolescent's pregnancy.
- Help the family explore previously successful coping mechanisms.
- Assist with development of a plan to deal with the pregnancy; encourage discussion of future plans.
- Encourage involvement of the adolescent's partner if she and the family desire.
- Reinforce the family members' understanding of the adolescent's need for their support, and teach ways that they can be supportive.

NURSING DIAGNOSIS

Ineffective management of therapeutic regimen related to inadequate knowledge of prenatal care and inconsistent participation in it

DESIRED PATIENT OUTCOME

The patient will knowledgeably manage her therapeutic regimen and consistently participate in prenatal care

Outcome measurement criteria

☐ Attendance at all scheduled prenatal visits

☐ Verbalization of correct dietary and exercise requirements during pregnancy

☐ Report of appropriate dietary intake

☐ Appropriate weight gain

☐ Participation in a daily moderate exercise program

☐ Verbalization of an understanding of risks associated with adolescent pregnancy

☐ Verbalization of an understanding of signs and symptoms of complications

☐ Verbalization of the need to notify a health care professional if signs of complications occur

☐ Verbalization of accurate knowledge of safe use of medications, if prescribed

☐ Appropriate use of medications, if prescribed, during pregnancy

Key interventions

- Assess the patient's ability to attend prenatal visits. Arrange for transportation or other assistance as needed.

- Emphasize the importance of prenatal monitoring and strongly encourage the patient to receive all prenatal care.

- Maintain an accepting, nonthreatening manner. For example, offer choices rather than make demands and encourage the patient to participate in her care.

- Assess the patient's knowledge of the importance of appropriate diet and exercise during pregnancy. Help her evaluate her typical diet and exercise patterns.

- Teach the patient about specific dietary requirements during pregnancy. Refer her to a nutritionist if needed.

- Teach the patient about normal weight gain during pregnancy. Evaluate and document her weight at each prenatal visit.

- Encourage participation in safe, regular exercise.

- Discuss common risks associated with adolescent pregnancy: low-birth-weight infant, pregnancy-induced hypertension (PIH), and preterm labor.

- Describe signs and symptoms of PIH and preterm labor. Emphasize the need to notify a health care professional if signs and symptoms occur.

- Explain the safe use of prescribed medications, including their dosages, benefits, and adverse effects. Discuss how to manage adverse effects. Also, stress the need to avoid using over-the-counter or other medications that have not been prescribed specifically for her.

- Reinforce the need to avoid alcohol and all illicit drugs.

- Stress the importance of self-care between visits. At subsequent visits, reassess the patient's need for further instructions about self-care.

- Supplement teaching sessions with written information appropriate for the patient's reading level.

NURSING DIAGNOSIS

High risk for altered parenting related to inadequate support systems, lack of knowledge, and unrealistic expectations

DESIRED PATIENT OUTCOME

The patient will manage parenting activities effectively and safely

Outcome measurement criteria

☐ Verbalization of concerns about parenting

☐ Use of appropriate resources to learn parenting skills

☐ Use of appropriate resources to increase knowledge about infant behavior and development

☐ Identification of personal difficulties with parenting

☐ Participation in problem solving to address concerns about parenting

☐ Demonstration of safe, effective parenting skills

Key interventions

- Assess the patient's plans for infant care. Help her explore her attitudes about parenting. Be alert for lack of realism about the abilities of infants.

- Encourage the patient to spend time with people who have infants and discuss concerns about parenting.

- Refer the patient to resources for learning parenting skills. Encourage her to discuss feelings about new information.

- Provide information about normal pediatric growth and development. Encourage the patient to compare her expectations to this information.

- Help the patient plan safe, effective ways to deal with parenting difficulties. Re-evaluate her parenting skills periodically.

Advanced maternal age during pregnancy

Pregnancy in a woman over age 35.

NURSING DIAGNOSIS

Altered family processes related to integration of the expected infant into established patterns of family functioning

DESIRED PATIENT OUTCOME

The patient's family will adapt successfully to changes in family processes created by the expected infant

Outcome measurement criteria

☐ Verbalization of feelings about integrating the expected infant

☐ Development of plans for successful integration of the expected infant

☐ Verbalization of adaptation to anticipated changes in family processes

Key interventions

• Encourage family members to explore anticipated changes and express feelings about the effects of pregnancy and the expected infant on family functioning. Encourage open communication among family members and health care professionals.

• Help family members examine daily activities and plan to include the infant in them. Encourage discussion of such topics as division of tasks and alternate ways to meet family members' needs.

- Encourage family members to recognize the potential effect of pregnancy and child care on the mother's energy level. Also help them plan strategies to deal with the infant's and family's needs.

- Encourage the parents to plan to protect their relationship as a couple. Recommend scheduling occasional time away from the infant to maintain relationship integrity.

NURSING DIAGNOSIS

Health-seeking behaviors (appropriate self-care) related to involvement in the therapeutic regimen during pregnancy

DESIRED PATIENT OUTCOME

The patient will remain involved in health maintenance throughout pregnancy

Outcome measurement criteria

- ☐ Compliance with scheduled antepartal visits with health care professionals
- ☐ Maintenance of appropriate diet, exercise, and rest regimens
- ☐ Appropriate use of medication, if prescribed
- ☐ Participation in decision making about recommended diagnostic tests

Key interventions

- Assess the patient's knowledge of prenatal care and teach about scheduled visits.
- Assess the patient's knowledge of diet, exercise, and rest requirements during pregnancy. Provide information as needed and correct any misconceptions.

- Assess the patient's knowledge of appropriate use of medications, if prescribed during pregnancy. Teach her about each medication's dosage schedule, therapeutic effects, adverse effects, and potential interactions with other drugs or food.

- Teach the patient about recommended diagnostic tests; involve her in decisions about testing.

Anemia

Below-normal hemoglobin level, hematocrit, or both.

NURSING DIAGNOSIS

Altered nutrition: less than body requirements, related to inadequate iron intake and increased need for iron

DESIRED PATIENT OUTCOME

The patient will consume sufficient dietary and supplemental iron

Outcome measurement criteria

☐ Hemoglobin and hematocrit values within normal limits for pregnancy

☐ Correct identification of risks associated with anemia during pregnancy

☐ Verbalization of accurate knowledge of the safe, effective use of supplemental iron

☐ Correct identification of iron-rich foods

Key interventions

- Obtain hemoglobin and hematocrit values, as prescribed. Explain their significance to the patient.

- Describe the risks of anemia during pregnancy: fatigue, infection, pregnancy-induced hypertension, premature delivery, low-birth-weight infant, postpartal hemorrhage, and delayed healing.

- Explain the need for increased iron during pregnancy and the difficulty in meeting this need through diet alone.

- Teach about iron-rich foods and encourage their consumption.

- Teach about supplemental iron therapy. Explain that the stool color normally changes to black during such therapy.

- Explain the need to increase fluid and fiber intake during supplemental iron therapy to avoid constipation.

- Stress the need to keep iron supplements away from children; accidental ingestion may be lethal.

- Explain that vitamin C increases absorption of supplemental iron. Encourage increased intake of foods high in vitamin C.

- Explain that supplemental iron absorption is decreased somewhat when taken with food, but that GI discomfort may occur if iron is taken on an empty stomach. Teach the patient to take iron at bedtime or shortly after meals if GI discomfort occurs.

Cervical incompetence

Painless, spontaneous, premature dilation of the cervical os, especially during the second trimester.

NURSING DIAGNOSIS

Anxiety related to unknown pregnancy outcome secondary to cervical incompetence

DESIRED PATIENT OUTCOME

The patient and family will manage anxiety effectively and report confidence in coping with an unknown pregnancy outcome

Outcome measurement criteria

☐ Verbalization of accurate knowledge of the therapeutic regimen

☐ Demonstration of effective anxiety-reducing techniques

☐ Report of anxiety reduction to a tolerable level

☐ Identification of danger signs of inevitable abortion, infection, premature rupture of membranes (PROM), and preterm labor

☐ Expression of confidence in the ability to follow the treatment plan

Key interventions

• Assess the patient's and family's anxiety level. Provide a supportive atmosphere and establish therapeutic relationships.

• Assess the patient's and family's knowledge of the condition. Clarify any misconceptions, using short, simple sentences during episodes of acute anxiety.

- Provide more detailed information as the patient and family indicate a readiness to discuss causes of cervical incompetence and the benefits and risks of various treatment options.

- Encourage the patient and family to verbalize feelings about the condition and its treatment.

- Monitor fetal heart tones and assess for uterine contractions. As appropriate, reassure the patient and family about fetal well-being and let them listen to fetal heart tones.

- Teach the patient and family to recognize the signs of inevitable abortion, infection, PROM, and preterm labor. Instruct them to report such warning signs and symptoms as contractions, cramps, oral temperature above 100° F (37° C), and clear or bloody vaginal fluid.

- Teach self-monitoring methods, including palpating for contractions and counting fetal kicks.

- Help the patient and family identify previously successful methods for coping with anxiety. Encourage them to use these methods and suggest alternative methods as needed.

- Help the patient and family develop a plan of action when anxiety is overwhelming, which may include mobilizing family support, seeking counseling, and contacting a health care professional.

Diabetes mellitus

An endocrine disorder of metabolism that may occur before pregnancy or may be limited to glucose intolerance during pregnancy (gestational diabetes).

NURSING DIAGNOSIS

Fear related to the effects of diabetes on maternal and fetal well-being

DESIRED PATIENT OUTCOME

The patient will express decreased fear about the actual and potential effects of diabetes

Outcome measurement criteria

☐ Verbalization of specific concerns about personal and fetal effects

☐ Use of effective coping mechanisms to deal with fears

☐ Participation in problem solving related to care

Key interventions

• Establish a therapeutic relationship with the patient. Encourage her to express feelings about the disorder and specific concerns about its effects.

• Give the patient accurate, complete information to address questions, concerns, or fears.

• Help the patient identify previously successful techniques for coping with stressful situations.

• Help the patient become involved in problem solving related to managing her pregnancy. Praise her efforts to become active in problem solving.

• Reassess the patient's feelings during follow-up visits. Refer her to counselors, clergy, or support groups as needed.

NURSING DIAGNOSIS

Ineffective management of therapeutic regimen related to lack of knowledge about and complexity of the regimen

DESIRED PATIENT OUTCOME

The patient will manage the therapeutic regimen successfully throughout her pregnancy

Outcome measurement criteria

☐ Verbalization of knowledge of basic pathophysiology of diabetes mellitus

☐ Verbalization of understanding of and adherence to the prescribed diet

☐ Verbalization of an accurate understanding of the relation between rest, exercise, and blood glucose regulation

☐ Verbalization of correct knowledge of safe use of insulin

☐ Demonstration of safe self-administration of insulin

☐ Verbalization of the risk of pregnancy complications caused by diabetes mellitus

☐ Correct identification of signs and symptoms of complications

☐ Proper use of self-care measures if complications occur

☐ Expression of confidence in ability to manage the therapeutic regimen

☐ Report of use of effective techniques to manage diet, rest, and exercise

☐ Weight gain within normal limits for pregnancy

☐ Blood glucose level within normal limits

Key interventions

- Assess the patient's understanding of diabetes. Using language and terms appropriate to her level of understanding, explain the disorder's basic pathophysiology, the need to control the blood glucose level, and the methods used to control it.

- Assess the patient's understanding of the prescribed diet. As needed, refer her to a nutritionist or support group for help with diet management.

- Assess the patient's usual level of rest and exercise. Teach her about the relation between exercise and diet in regulating blood glucose.

- Help the patient develop a plan to comply with the prescribed rest, exercise, and diet regimen.

- Stress the importance of proper insulin use and regular blood glucose monitoring.

- Assess the patient's knowledge and use of insulin and any other prescribed medications. Teach about appropriate dosage, self-administration, benefits, and adverse effects.

- Assess the patient's knowledge of diabetes-related risks during pregnancy, such as pregnancy-induced hypertension (PIH), preterm labor, and macrosomia.

- Stress the need for careful monitoring during pregnancy. Explain pertinent diagnostic and laboratory tests.

- Describe the signs and symptoms of preterm labor and PIH.

- Stress the importance of regular prenatal care and strict adherence to the care plan. Explain that the care plan may change throughout pregnancy as metabolic needs change.

- Verify the patient's confidence in managing self-care. Help her develop the skills needed to perform self-care, especially self-care for complications.

- Teach the patient how to monitor her blood glucose level and weight. Document periodic weight measurements and assist with blood glucose evaluation as prescribed.

- Teach the patient about the need for periodic blood glucose evaluations after pregnancy. Inform her of the incidence (40%) of continued diabetes after delivery.

NURSING DIAGNOSIS

High risk for injury related to unstable blood glucose level

DESIRED PATIENT OUTCOME

The patient will remain free from injury caused by hyperglycemia or hypoglycemia

Outcome measurement criteria

☐ Verbalization of correct signs and symptoms of hyperglycemia and hypoglycemia

☐ Verbalization of appropriate self-treatment of hyperglycemia and hypoglycemia

☐ Verbalization and use of safe techniques to avoid or manage hyperglycemia and hypoglycemia

Key interventions

- Assess the patient's knowledge of the risks of hyperglycemia and hypoglycemia in pregnancy. Provide accurate information to increase knowledge and correct misconceptions.

- Describe the signs of hyperglycemia, such as thirst, nausea, vomiting, abdominal pain, increased urination, drowsiness, flushed skin, and weak, rapid pulse; and hypoglycemia, such as hunger, sweating, fatigue, weakness, nervousness, dizziness, headache, and pallor.

- Teach about effective self-treatment of hyperglycemia, such as self-administration of insulin, and hypoglycemia, such as immediate consumption of fruit juice, hard candy, honey, or other carbohydrate.

- Teach a family member how to administer oral glucose and glucagon to the patient.

Discomforts of the first trimester

Common alterations in well-being during early pregnancy, including nausea, vomiting, urinary frequency and urgency, fatigue, headache, and sexual concerns.

NURSING DIAGNOSIS

Altered nutrition: less than body requirements, related to nausea and vomiting in early pregnancy

DESIRED PATIENT OUTCOME

The patient will consume sufficient nutrients to support herself and the fetus

Outcome measurement criteria

☐ Verbalization of understanding of appropriate ways to avoid nausea and vomiting

☐ Verbalization of the need for adequate caloric intake to support pregnancy

☐ Maintenance of prepregnancy weight or 2- to 5-lb (0.9- to 2.2-kg) increase during the first trimester

☐ Decreased frequency of nausea and vomiting

☐ Consumption of an adequate, appropriate diet

Key interventions

• Assess the frequency and severity of nausea and vomiting.

• Recommend ways to help decrease nausea and vomiting, such as decreasing exposure to noxious odors, arising slowly from bed, avoiding sudden movements, and walking outdoors.

- Recommend dietary practices to decrease nausea and vomiting, such as eating one or two crackers before arising from bed, avoiding fried foods, drinking liquids between meals instead of with meals, eating several small meals a day rather than a few large meals, drinking herbal tea, and eating high-protein food and fruit to avoid hypoglycemia.

- Help the patient plan to consume 2,200 to 2,500 calories per day. Evaluate a 24-hour diet history and discuss the strengths and weaknesses of the patient's dietary choices. Refer her to a dietitian as needed.

- Assess the incidence of nausea and vomiting during follow-up visits.

- Document the patient's weight at each visit.

NURSING DIAGNOSIS

Altered urinary elimination related to urinary frequency and urgency caused by the physiologic changes that occur during early pregnancy

DESIRED PATIENT OUTCOME

The patient will maintain appropriate urinary elimination patterns

Outcome measurement criteria

☐ Verbalization of effective urination control methods

☐ Verbalization of effective techniques to decrease nocturia and urine leakage

Key interventions

- Assess the patient's urinary elimination pattern. Discuss the increased frequency and urgency commonly associated with pregnancy.

- Recommend ways to decrease nocturia, such as decreasing liquid intake at night, avoiding caffeine, and voiding immediately before bedtime.
- Teach pelvic floor exercises to increase muscle tone and decrease stress incontinence.

NURSING DIAGNOSIS

High risk for infection related to the physiologic effects of pregnancy on the urinary tract

DESIRED PATIENT OUTCOME

The patient will remain free from urinary tract infection (UTI) throughout pregnancy

Outcome measurement criteria

- ☐ Verbalization of the increased risk of UTI during pregnancy
- ☐ Correct identification of signs and symptoms of UTI
- ☐ Verbalization of effective UTI management
- ☐ Verbalization of understanding of the need for prompt, effective treatment of UTI during pregnancy
- ☐ Absence of signs and symptoms of UTI

Key interventions

- Explain the increased risk of UTI during pregnancy because of anatomic and hormonal changes.
- Teach hygiene measures that help prevent UTI, such as wiping from front to back after urination or defecation, using new tissue for each wipe, avoiding tight-fitting garments, avoiding plastic-backed panty liners, wearing cotton undergarments, and sleeping without underclothes.

- Describe the signs and symptoms of UTI, including urinary frequency and urgency, burning on urination, bladder discomfort, and bladder spasm on urination. Instruct the patient to report them if they occur.
- Explain that untreated UTI during pregnancy may trigger preterm labor.

NURSING DIAGNOSIS

Fatigue related to the increased physiologic demands of early pregnancy

DESIRED PATIENT OUTCOME

The patient will decrease fatigue by managing activities judiciously

Outcome measurement criteria

- ☐ Report of increased rest periods during the day
- ☐ Report of increased sleep at night
- ☐ Description of schedule alterations that include adequate rest periods
- ☐ Report and documentation of adequate nutritional intake
- ☐ Verbalization of decreased fatigue

Key interventions

- Assess the patient's sleep and rest patterns. Encourage her to pay attention to her need for rest and to avoid extreme fatigue.
- Help the patient examine her daily schedule and adjust it to include rest periods. Encourage her to sit with her feet propped up several times a day. Recommend daytime naps if needed.

- Recommend pacing of activities throughout the day to avoid fatigue.

- Encourage the patient and her partner to divide household chores and child care duties as needed to provide more time for rest.

- Encourage retiring earlier in the evening to increase total sleep time.

- Encourage appropriate dietary intake for physiologic support. Recommend regular exercise.

NURSING DIAGNOSIS

Altered sexuality patterns related to pregnancy discomforts and fear about the effects of sexual activity on the fetus

DESIRED PATIENT OUTCOME

The patient will express satisfaction with sexual interactions

Outcome measurement criteria

☐ Sharing of concerns about the effects of sexual activity on the fetus

☐ Verbalization of an accurate understanding of fetal risks of sexual activity

☐ Identification of safe sexual practices during pregnancy

☐ Verbalization of the effect of pregnancy on sexual drive

☐ Report of accurate knowledge of various means of sexual expression

☐ Verbalization of satisfaction with sexual expression during pregnancy

Key interventions

- Establish a rapport with the patient. Encourage open discussion of concerns related to sexual activity during pregnancy.

- Provide accurate information about sexual activity during pregnancy. Reassure the patient that, in the absence of certain risk factors, intercourse is safe during pregnancy.

- Encourage the patient and her partner to communicate their sexual needs.

- Assess the patient's risk for sexually transmitted diseases. Discuss and encourage safe-sex practices.

- Explain that women may experience increased—or decreased—sexual drive during pregnancy. Some women note decreased sexual drive during the first and third trimesters and increased drive during the second trimester; others note a gradual decrease in drive as pregnancy progresses.

- Encourage the patient and her partner to explore alternate methods of achieving sexual satisfaction. Caution against inserting objects into the vagina or blowing air into the vagina.

- Encourage exploration of various positions for intercourse as pregnancy progresses. Explain that women should avoid the supine position during the third trimester to decrease the risk of supine hypotension.

- Evaluate the patient's feelings about sexual satisfaction during follow-up visits.

NURSING DIAGNOSIS

Pain related to headaches caused by the physiologic effects of early pregnancy

DESIRED PATIENT OUTCOME
The patient will manage headache pain effectively

Outcome measurement criteria
☐ Correct identification of the causes of headaches

☐ Use of an effective plan to manage headaches

☐ Verbalization of danger signs associated with headaches

☐ Report of tolerance of headaches

☐ Absence or reduction in the number of headaches

Key interventions
- Assess the location, precipitating factors, and severity of the patient's headaches. Determine whether the headaches are typical for her.

- Explain that headaches may result from increased blood volume during pregnancy, fatigue, or emotional stress.

- Assess for nasal stuffiness and epistaxis and explain that these are common causes of headaches during pregnancy.

- Teach the patient to avoid headaches by obtaining sufficient sleep and rest, eating regularly, drinking sufficient fluids, avoiding smoke-filled environments, and avoiding known and suspected allergens.

- Recommend nonpharmacologic methods of treating headache, such as applying cool, wet cloths to the forehead and neck, using relaxation exercises, massaging the back and neck, taking a warm bath or shower, walking slowly in the fresh air, breathing steam in the bathroom, and using a cool mist vaporizer.

- Stress the need to consult a health care professional before taking an over-the-counter or prescription headache medication.

- Instruct the patient to recognize and report danger signs associated with headaches during pregnancy: severe, frequent, or long-lasting headaches; blurred vision; and edema of the face, hands, and legs in the morning.
- Assess the incidence of headaches and the effectiveness of their management during follow-up visits.

NURSING DIAGNOSIS

High risk for injury related to frequent dizziness and fainting caused by the effects of early pregnancy

DESIRED PATIENT OUTCOME

The patient will remain free from injury caused by dizziness or fainting

Outcome measurement criteria

☐ Correct identification of factors that cause dizziness and fainting
☐ Verbalization of effective ways to minimize dizziness and fainting
☐ Verbalization of effective ways to manage fainting episodes
☐ Report of decreased frequency of dizziness and fainting

Key interventions

- Assess episodes of dizziness and fainting to determine their frequency, precipitating factors, and relation to nausea, vomiting, activity, and time of day.
- Teach the patient that dizziness and fainting are common in pregnancy and may be caused by physiologic changes of pregnancy, inadequate diet, acute illness, or extreme anxiety.

- Recommend minimizing dizziness and fainting by rising slowly from a sitting or lying position, resting in a lateral rather than supine position, resting frequently throughout the day, eating small frequent meals rather than a few large meals, and avoiding overexertion.

- Teach the patient to manage episodes of fainting and dizziness by sitting down or lying on her left side. Encourage her to notify a health care professional if fainting results in a fall.

- Assess for recurrence of dizziness and fainting on follow-up visits.

Discomforts of the second trimester

Common alterations in well-being during advancing pregnancy, including heartburn, constipation, varicosities, hemorrhoids, and supine hypotension.

NURSING DIAGNOSIS

Pain related to heartburn, varicosities, or hemorrhoids caused by the physiologic changes of pregnancy

DESIRED PATIENT OUTCOME

The patient will use pain-relief measures and report decreased pain

Outcome measurement criteria

☐ Correct identification of the causes of pain

☐ Verbalization of appropriate methods to avoid and manage pain

☐ Effective use of pharmacologic and nonpharmacologic pain-relief techniques

☐ Report of no discomfort or pain

Key interventions

• Assess for pain associated with heartburn, varicosities, or hemorrhoids. Teach about the physiologic changes of pregnancy that increase the incidence of these problems.

• Teach the patient how to prevent heartburn by decreasing her intake of fried foods; avoiding highly spiced foods, foods known to cause indigestion, and coffee; eating several small meals instead of a few large meals; avoiding tight clothing; drinking several glasses of water per day; and sitting upright after meals.

- Teach the patient to manage heartburn by sleeping on several pillows, sipping carbonated beverages, eating a small serving of yogurt, or taking an antacid with an aluminum salt base whenever the pain occurs.

- Instruct the patient to prevent varicosities by exercising regularly, avoiding clothes that fit tightly on the legs, wearing full-length support hose when standing or walking for long periods, avoiding long periods of sitting or standing, and wearing well-padded shoes.

- Teach her to manage the pain of varicosities by elevating her legs above heart level when pain occurs, lying on the floor and propping her extended legs on a wall in the evenings, and wearing support hose.

- Instruct the patient to prevent hemorrhoids by not delaying bowel movements, not sitting on the toilet for long periods, not straining when defecating, drinking 8 to 10 glasses of water per day, increasing dietary fiber intake, and doing Kegel exercises regularly.

- Teach her to manage the pain of hemorrhoids by lying in a knee-chest position for 15 minutes when pain is acute, sitting in a warm tub, and using witch hazel compresses.

- Evaluate for successful management of heartburn, varicosities, and hemorrhoids during follow-up visits.

NURSING DIAGNOSIS

Constipation related to the physiologic changes of pregnancy and painful hemorrhoids

DESIRED PATIENT OUTCOME

The patient will resume normal bowel activity with no pain on defecation

Outcome measurement criteria

☐ Correct identification of the physiologic changes of pregnancy that contribute to constipation

☐ Verbalization and use of safe methods to decrease constipation

☐ Report of decreased constipation

Key interventions

• Assess the patient's understanding of the causes of constipation. Explain the physiologic effects of pregnancy that cause constipation.

• Instruct the patient to avoid constipation by increasing fluid intake, exercising regularly, not delaying bowel movements, elevating her feet on a stool in front of the toilet to achieve a squatting position, and increasing dietary fiber by eating more fruits, vegetables, and whole-grain bread and cereal.

• Teach about safe use of prescribed medications, such as stool softeners. Instruct the patient to avoid strong laxatives and to consult a health care professional before taking any medication, including over-the-counter medication.

• Assess for successful management of constipation during follow-up visits.

NURSING DIAGNOSIS

High risk for injury (fetal or maternal) related to the effects of supine hypotension

DESIRED PATIENT OUTCOME

The patient and fetus will remain free from injury related to supine hypotension during pregnancy

Outcome measurement criteria

☐ Correct identification of the causes and risks of supine hypotension

☐ Verbalization of effective methods to avoid supine hypotension

Key interventions

• Assess episodes of supine hypotension. Teach the patient about its causes.

• Explain that supine hypotension can decrease placental perfusion and blood circulation to the fetus.

• Teach the patient to avoid supine hypotension by assuming a side-lying or semi-Fowler's position rather than lying supine. Recommend that she elevate her upper body with pillows to keep the weight of the uterus off the vena cava.

• Assess for recurring episodes of supine hypotension during follow-up visits.

Discomforts of the third trimester

Common alterations in well-being during advanced pregnancy, including round ligament pain, dyspnea, backache, leg cramps, perineal pressure, Braxton Hicks contractions, insomnia, and pedal edema.

NURSING DIAGNOSIS

Pain related to round ligament stretching, leg cramps, perineal pressure, Braxton Hicks contractions, or backache secondary to advanced pregnancy

DESIRED PATIENT OUTCOME

The patient will successfully manage the pain associated with advanced pregnancy and will report decreased pain

Outcome measurement criteria

☐ Correct identification of causes of pain

☐ Verbalization of effective ways to prevent or manage pain

☐ Use of safe methods to manage pain

☐ Report of no discomfort or pain

Key interventions

• Teach the patient about the causes of her pain. Assess the nature of the pain and evaluate for potential complications, such as preterm labor.

• Instruct the patient to minimize round ligament pain by resting sufficiently, avoiding rapid twisting motions, rising slowly from a recumbent position, and avoiding excessive walking, standing, and exercising.

- Teach the patient to manage round ligament pain by applying heat to the affected area, performing total body relaxation exercises, and assuming a squatting or knee-chest position.

- Instruct the patient to prevent leg cramps by consuming adequate (but not excessive) dairy products, keeping her legs warm, avoiding toe-pointing during exercise or stretching, and taking a warm bath at bedtime.

- Teach her to manage leg cramps by walking, standing and leaning forward on the affected leg, dorsiflexing the foot with the knee extended, applying heat, and taking a warm bath.

- Instruct the patient to prevent excessive perineal pressure by resting sufficiently, avoiding excessive walking or standing, maintaining good body mechanics and posture, and wearing a maternity girdle.

- Teach her to manage perineal pressure by performing Kegel exercises and resting in a lateral position.

- Instruct the patient to prevent Braxton Hicks contractions by avoiding excessive physical activity. Teach her how to distinguish between Braxton Hicks contractions and true labor. Explain the risks of preterm labor and tell her to contact a health care professional immediately if signs of preterm labor occur.

- Teach her to manage Braxton Hicks contractions by walking if contractions occur during rest, resting if contractions occur during activity, changing position, performing effleurage, and taking a warm shower or bath.

- Instruct the patient to prevent backache by resting frequently, avoiding fatigue and overexertion, exercising regularly, using good body mechanics when lifting, maintaining good posture, wearing flat shoes with good support, and avoiding excessive weight gain.

- Teach her to manage backache by performing pelvic tilt exercises, getting back rubs, performing relaxation exercises, sitting in the tailor position, and applying heat.

NURSING DIAGNOSIS

Activity intolerance related to dyspnea secondary to the physiologic effects of advanced pregnancy

DESIRED PATIENT OUTCOME

The patient will experience decreased activity intolerance and will alter activities to compensate for dyspnea

Outcome measurement criteria

☐ Correct identification of physiologic causes of activity intolerance

☐ Report of altered daily schedule to accommodate decreased ability to tolerate activity

☐ Report of frequent rest periods throughout the day

Key interventions

- Teach the patient about the physiologic changes that contribute to dyspnea.

- Encourage the patient to assess her activities of daily living and to explore ways to get more rest. Reassure her that activity intolerance is transient.

- Instruct the patient how to help prevent dyspnea by maintaining good posture, avoiding overeating, sleeping with her upper body propped on several pillows, and planning short periods of activity rather than extended ones.

- Tell her to notify a health care professional if she experiences extreme shortness of breath or difficulty resuming normal breathing after an episode of dyspnea.

NURSING DIAGNOSIS

Sleep pattern disturbance related to insomnia secondary to advanced pregnancy

DESIRED PATIENT OUTCOME

The patient will obtain adequate, restful sleep

Outcome measurement criteria

☐ Verbalization and use of safe methods of promoting sleep

☐ Report of avoiding unsafe methods of obtaining sleep

☐ Report of an adequate sleep pattern

Key interventions

- Teach the patient about safe methods to promote sleep, including taking a warm bath at bedtime; getting a back rub or performing effleurage; performing relaxation exercises; having a warm drink at bedtime; avoiding large meals and caffeine for 3 hours before bedtime; limiting naps during the day; using several pillows as needed to support the abdomen, separate the knees, and elevate the head; limiting stimulation; and decreasing fluid intake in the evening.

- Stress the importance of avoiding over-the-counter sleep aids or alcohol to induce sleep. Tell the patient to notify a health care professional if insomnia becomes extreme.

- Assess for recurrence or exacerbation of insomnia during follow-up visits.

NURSING DIAGNOSIS

Altered peripheral tissue perfusion related to edema caused by the physiologic effects of pregnancy

DESIRED PATIENT OUTCOME

The patient will manage peripheral edema effectively and will report decreased incidence of this condition

Outcome measurement criteria

☐ Accurate description of the physiologic effects of pregnancy that decrease venous return

☐ Correct identification of danger signs associated with peripheral edema

☐ Verbalization and use of appropriate ways to avoid and manage peripheral edema

Key interventions

- Assess the location and severity of edema. Explain the physiologic changes of pregnancy that increase the risk of peripheral edema.

- Teach the patient how to identify edema associated with pregnancy-induced hypertension (PIH). Specifically, have the patient check for ankle edema in the morning or after she has rested for many hours. Persistent edema may indicate PIH.

- Tell the patient to prevent or manage edema by elevating her legs for 15 to 20 minutes two or three times a day, limiting dietary sodium intake, increasing dietary protein intake, avoiding constrictive clothing around the legs, avoiding prolonged standing, and putting on support hose before arising from bed in the morning.

- Instruct the patient to avoid diuretics.

- Reassess for edema during follow-up visits.

Ectopic pregnancy

Implantation of a fertilized ovum outside the uterine cavity, most commonly in a fallopian tube.

NURSING DIAGNOSIS

Pain related to the effects of tubal rupture from ectopic pregnancy or surgery for it

DESIRED PATIENT OUTCOME

The patient will use effective pain-control methods and report decreased pain

Outcome measurement criteria

☐ Correct identification of pharmacologic and nonpharmacologic pain-control methods

☐ Absence of signs of pain

☐ Report of decreased pain

Key interventions

• Assess for verbal and nonverbal indications of pain. Ask the patient to rate the pain on a scale of 1 to 10 and identify where the pain is most intense.

• Teach the patient about causes of the pain (such as rupture, bleeding, or incision), plans to control pain, and methods to prevent pain, such as splinting the surgical incision and changing position.

• Explain the appropriate use, benefits, and adverse effects of prescribed pain medication. Reinforce the need to control pain rather than let it become so severe that it impairs her ability to ambulate, breathe deeply, and change position easily.

- Discuss and encourage the use of nonpharmacologic pain-relief methods, such as warm baths, back rubs, use of a heating pad or hot water bottle, and relaxation techniques.

NURSING DIAGNOSIS

Fluid volume deficit related to excessive fluid loss secondary to complications of ectopic pregnancy or surgery for it

DESIRED PATIENT OUTCOME

The patient will exhibit restored or stable circulating fluid volume

Outcome measurement criteria

☐ Absence of signs and symptoms of hypovolemia

☐ Vital signs within normal limits

☐ Laboratory values within normal limits

☐ Report of absence of vomiting

☐ Report of adequate fluid intake

Key interventions

- Monitor fluid intake and output, vital signs, and laboratory test results, as prescribed. Document the amount and character of fluid intake and output.

- Assess for signs and symptoms of hypovolemia, such as vertigo, hypotension, tachycardia, shoulder pain (if internal bleeding occurs), poor skin turgor, vomiting, decreased urine output, and abnormally low hemoglobin, hematocrit, and electrolyte values.

- Administer I.V. fluid or blood products as prescribed.

- Administer prescribed antiemetics.

- Offer various liquids by mouth as the patient can

tolerate. Encourage her to drink 8 to 10 glasses of fluid per day when nausea subsides.

NURSING DIAGNOSIS

High risk for dysfunctional grieving related to the effects of pregnancy loss or salpingectomy

DESIRED PATIENT OUTCOME

The patient and family will demonstrate progress through the stages of grief and realistic expectations for future pregnancies

Outcome measurement criteria

☐ Identification and expression of grief

☐ Participation in appropriate self-care activities

☐ Resumption of normal activities of daily living

☐ Verbalization of an accurate understanding of the impact of surgery on future pregnancies

Key interventions

- Establish a therapeutic relationship with the patient and family and validate their loss. When appropriate, discuss the stages of grief.

- Encourage the patient and family to discuss their feelings about the loss.

- Discuss differences in individual and cultural responses to grief. Explain that each family member will progress at his or her pace. Encourage open communication among family members.

- Teach the patient and family that emotional lability is normal after such a loss. Encourage them to be support-ive of one another.

- Help the patient perform self-care within the limits of

her activity tolerance. Describe the signs of wound healing so that she can evaluate her progress.

- Encourage the patient to obtain sufficient rest to promote physical and emotional recovery.

- Provide accurate information about ectopic pregnancy, including its impact on future pregnancies.

- Provide information about support groups, counselors, clergy, or telephone support, as needed. Encourage the use of these or other resources if depression or difficulty resolving grief occurs.

Elective termination of pregnancy

Deliberate interruption of an unwanted pregnancy before it is viable.

NURSING DIAGNOSIS

Decisional conflict related to ambivalence about pregnancy termination

DESIRED PATIENT OUTCOME

The patient will resolve decisional conflict and express satisfaction with her decision

Outcome measurement criteria

☐ Verbalization of accurate knowledge about available options

☐ Verbalization of each option's advantages and disadvantages to her

☐ Documentation of informed consent

☐ Report of satisfaction with her decision

Key interventions

• Provide information about available options for continuation or termination of the pregnancy based on the patient's preference, duration of pregnancy, and social situation.

• Provide information about psychological, social, and physical risks and benefits of abortion.

• Help the patient examine the positive and negative effects of abortion, adoption, or child-rearing on herself and others.

- Help the patient identify and explore personal fears or conflicts associated with various choices.

- Encourage the involvement of significant others in decision making as the patient desires, but reinforce that the decision is the patient's.

- Assist with documentation of informed consent as needed.

- Assess the patient's attitude toward her decision to terminate or continue the pregnancy. As needed, refer her to support groups, community agencies, and other sources of support.

NURSING DIAGNOSIS

Fear related to pregnancy-termination surgery and its implications for future pregnancies

DESIRED PATIENT OUTCOME

The patient will report decreased fear related to pregnancy-termination surgery and future childbearing

Outcome measurement criteria

☐ Verbalization of accurate knowledge about pregnancy-termination surgery

☐ Verbalization of correct understanding of typical physical and emotional recovery

☐ Verbalization of the need for effective contraception

☐ Demonstration and report of reduced fear

Key interventions

- Help the patient recognize her fears. Reassure her that fears are normal.

- Provide accurate information about the procedure, using simple, direct statements and avoiding excessive details.

- Discuss the normal course of physical recovery.

- Provide information about emotional recovery. Inform the patient that strong negative or positive feelings are common. Encourage her to contact support people during difficult times. Provide information about counseling services, as needed.

- Provide accurate information about the patient's ability to conceive in the future based on her situation.

- Stress the importance of using effective contraception with each episode of intercourse. Warn about the risk of becoming pregnant from unprotected intercourse before the next menses.

- Provide information about safe sex and contraceptive choices. Guide the patient to appropriate resources for obtaining contraceptive products and further information.

NURSING DIAGNOSIS

High risk for infection related to postoperative complications of elective termination of pregnancy

DESIRED PATIENT OUTCOME

The patient will not develop infection during recovery from pregnancy termination

Outcome measurement criteria

☐ Temperature within normal limits

☐ Absence of prolonged cramping, bleeding, and uterine tenderness

☐ Absence of foul-smelling vaginal bleeding or discharge

☐ Resumption of menstruation within 4 to 6 weeks

☐ Compliance with the postoperative plan of care

Key interventions

- Teach the patient to check her temperature twice daily for 1 week and to notify a health care professional if it exceeds 100° F (37° C).

- Explain normal postoperative bleeding. Describe it as typically similar to menses but possibly lighter or heavier and sometimes with brown or dark red clots. Note that spotting may occur for up to 1 month.

- Tell the patient to report heavy vaginal bleeding (bleeding that saturates more than two pads in 2 hours), bleeding that persists for more than 2 weeks, foul-smelling discharge, or passage of grayish clots.

- Explain that moderate cramping is normal but that severe or persistent cramping should be reported. Teach about nonpharmacologic relief measures, such as the use of lower abdominal massage and a heating pad or hot water bottle.

- Instruct the patient to introduce nothing into the vagina during the 1st week after the procedure to decrease the risk of infection. For example, tell her to avoid intercourse, tampons, and douching.

- Teach about prescribed medications, including their dosage schedule, benefits, and adverse effects. Reinforce the importance of completing the course of prescribed antibiotics.

- Encourage the patient to return for follow-up visits as recommended.

Human immunodeficiency virus infection

Seropositive state of a person infected with human immuno-deficiency virus (HIV), which eventually leads to immune system depression.

NURSING DIAGNOSIS

Ineffective individual coping related to difficulty accepting HIV-positive status

DESIRED PATIENT OUTCOME

The patient will cope with the diagnosis and verbalize knowledge of the effects of the disease

Outcome measurement criteria

☐ Verbalization of feelings related to HIV-positive status

☐ Identification of effective and ineffective coping mechanisms

☐ Use of effective coping mechanisms and avoidance of ineffective ones

☐ Identification of options to deal with the pregnancy

☐ Use of various resources for information and support

Key interventions

- Establish a therapeutic relationship with the patient. Accept the patient's initial reaction and adjust teaching plans according to her readiness to learn.

- Encourage the patient and family to discuss feelings related to her HIV status; maintain open communication so that she continues to feel free to express herself.

- Help the patient identify previously effective and ineffective coping mechanisms. Encourage her to use the effective ones.

- Discuss alternate coping mechanisms as needed, including relaxation, visualization, information gathering, use of support groups, and participation as a support person.

- Help the patient explore options for dealing with HIV infection during pregnancy. Offer information about treatment options and prognosis as the patient indicates readiness to learn. Also offer information about pregnancy termination and sterilization, if the patient expresses interest.

- Help the patient develop a plan for coping with other stressors. Refer her to support groups, information sources, counselors, social services, community agencies, or chemical dependency treatment units as needed.

- Schedule follow-up appointments as needed to meet the patient's needs.

NURSING DIAGNOSIS

Ineffective management of therapeutic regimen related to lack of knowledge and skill to manage the HIV infection, medication regimen, and infection control

DESIRED PATIENT OUTCOME

The patient will manage her treatment regimen effectively, using appropriate knowledge and skills

Outcome measurement criteria

☐ Verbalization of accurate knowledge about dietary management

☐ Active participation in the treatment regimen

☐ Maintenance of current weight or weight gain during pregnancy

☐ Correct identification of risk factors associated with disease transmission

☐ Use of techniques to decrease the risk of disease transmission

☐ Accurate description of the prescribed medication regimen

Key interventions

- Assess the patient's understanding of proper dietary intake during pregnancy and ability to obtain adequate food.

- Explain the increased dietary requirements during pregnancy. Stress the need for adequate nutrition to support the patient's compromised immune system.

- Provide nutritional counseling and refer her to community resources for dietary support as needed.

- Weigh the patient at each follow-up visit and document findings. Encourage her to monitor her weight.

- Suggest eating small, frequent meals to help minimize nausea and vomiting.

- Assess the patient's sleep, rest, and exercise patterns. Evaluate her ability to obtain adequate sleep, rest, and exercise. Help her develop a plan to support her immune system by obtaining adequate activity and rest.

- Assess the patient's knowledge about behaviors that increase the risk for HIV transmission. Encourage her to identify her behaviors that pose a high risk for transmission; discuss her sexual practices, drug use, and history of blood infusions. Help her develop a plan for decreasing the risk of further exposure of herself and others.

- Teach about the safe use of prescribed medications, including the dosage schedule, benefits, and adverse effects.

- Encourage the patient to keep all follow-up appointments.

NURSING DIAGNOSIS

High risk for infection related to decreased resistance secondary to immune system compromise by HIV infection

DESIRED PATIENT OUTCOME

The patient will remain free from opportunistic infection during pregnancy

Outcome measurement criteria

☐ Correct identification of ways to avoid infection

☐ Report of use of techniques to avoid infection

☐ Absence of signs and symptoms of infection

Key interventions

- Teach the patient to recognize and report signs and symptoms of infection, including fever, nausea, vomiting, fatigue, vaginal discharge, and cough.

- Explain health maintenance and hygiene practices that decrease the risk of opportunistic infection. Encourage appropriate diet, rest, sleep, exercise, and hygiene.

- Discuss the implications of immune system compromise. Tell the patient to limit contact with ill people in social or work settings.

- Take universal precautions and use appropriate techniques for hygiene and sanitation in the hospital. Use strict sterile technique for all invasive procedures.

- Monitor vital signs and overall physical status for signs of infection.

NURSING DIAGNOSIS

Hopelessness related to the terminal nature of HIV infection

DESIRED PATIENT OUTCOME

The patient will engage actively in self-care and will report confidence in her ability to cope with effects of the HIV infection

Outcome measurement criteria

☐ Verbalization of feelings about the future

☐ Use of safe, effective coping mechanisms to counteract feelings of hopelessness

☐ Participation in self-care and activities of daily living

☐ Participation in diversional activities

☐ Report of use of available resources as needed

Key interventions

• Assess the patient's and family's verbal and nonverbal responses to the diagnosis of HIV infection.

• Assess the patient's level of hopelessness. Be alert for defensive coping, inappropriate denial, and unsafe or ineffective coping mechanisms.

• Establish a rapport with the patient. Provide a safe atmosphere for open expression of feelings. Encourage exploration of the impact of HIV infection on future plans.

• Encourage exploration of specific factors that contribute to hopelessness. Help the patient develop a plan to cope with specific concerns.

• Urge the patient to explore previous experiences of hopelessness and discuss previously successful coping mechanisms. Help her develop a plan to deal with hopelessness.

- Assess the patient's available support systems. Encourage her to seek support during episodes of acute hopelessness. Involve support people in the patient's plan of care as she desires.

- Encourage the patient to participate in the plan of care for the present and future. Explain all tests, treatment options, and other aspects of care.

- Refer the patient to community resources, such as support groups, clergy, and information sources, as indicated. Encourage her to seek external support as needed.

NURSING DIAGNOSIS

High risk for infection (fetal) related to HIV exposure from the mother

DESIRED PATIENT OUTCOME

The patient will minimize the risk of HIV transmission to her fetus

Outcome measurement criteria

☐ Correct identification of danger signs during pregnancy

☐ Verbalization of ways to help prevent HIV transmission to the fetus

Key interventions

- Teach the patient to recognize and report danger signs, such as preterm labor, bleeding during pregnancy, and absence of fetal movement.

- Explain how to recognize membrane rupture; stress the need to immediately report spontaneous rupture of membranes.

- For related information, see "Infections" in the Intrapartal Period section.

Hyperemesis gravidarum

Excessive, persistent vomiting during pregnancy.

NURSING DIAGNOSIS

Altered nutrition: less than body requirements, related to abnormal fluid loss caused by hyperemesis gravidarum

DESIRED PATIENT OUTCOME

The patient will obtain sufficient dietary intake for adequate nutrition during pregnancy

Outcome measurement criteria

☐ Vital signs within normal limits

☐ Absence of signs of dehydration

☐ Urine output of more than 30 ml/hour

☐ Urine specific gravity of 1.010 to 1.025

☐ Electrolyte levels within normal limits

☐ Absence of vomiting

☐ Stabilization and eventual increase of weight

☐ Oral intake of at least 2,500 calories/day

☐ Fetal growth within normal limits

Key interventions

- Monitor vital signs, weight, skin turgor, mucous membrane moisture, and capillary refill time.
- Weigh the patient daily and record the weight.
- Monitor laboratory test results as indicated.
- Restrict the patient's oral intake as prescribed during acute hyperemesis gravidarum.

- Offer frequent small amounts of clear liquid or dry food when the patient can tolerate oral intake. Gradually increase oral intake as prescribed.

- Administer I.V. fluids, antiemetics, sedatives, and dietary supplements as prescribed. Explain the benefits and adverse effects of all medications.

- Provide the opportunity for regular oral hygiene.

- Monitor fluid intake and output carefully, particularly noting the amount and character of output.

- Investigate factors that seem to precipitate vomiting, such as odors or stress. Help the patient eliminate these factors from her environment.

- Teach the patient about appropriate nutrition during pregnancy, including calorie requirements and recommended intake of various foods and fluids. Provide written information for use at home.

- Assess and record fetal heart rate and fetal growth as ordered.

- Refer the patient for nutritional counseling.

NURSING DIAGNOSIS
Activity intolerance related to inadequate nutrition and fluid and electrolyte imbalance

DESIRED PATIENT OUTCOME
The patient will resume her prepregnancy level of activity tolerance

Outcome measurement criteria
☐ Absence of signs of activity intolerance
☐ Correct identification of factors that indicate reduced activity tolerance

☐ Alteration of daily schedule to allow frequent rest periods

☐ Report of tolerance of normal activities of daily living

Key interventions

- Assess for signs and symptoms of activity intolerance: weak or rapid pulse, dyspnea on exertion, shortness of breath, blood pressure changes, and reports of dizziness with normal activity.

- Teach the patient how to assess herself for signs and symptoms of activity intolerance. Urge her to limit activity when signs and symptoms occur.

- Encourage frequent rest periods during the day. Schedule care to decrease the number of disturbances for a hospitalized patient. Involve the patient in planning rest periods during hospitalization and at home.

- Help the patient gradually increase activity in the hospital and at home. During the acute phase, gradually increase the patient's participation in self-care activities.

NURSING DIAGNOSIS

Fear related to the effects of hyperemesis gravidarum on maternal and fetal well-being

DESIRED PATIENT OUTCOME

The patient and family will demonstrate effective coping with fears

Outcome measurement criteria

☐ Expression of specific fears about hyperemesis gravidarum

☐ Verbalization of accurate knowledge about potential effects of the disorder on the patient and fetus

☐ Demonstration of appropriate problem-solving behaviors to manage concerns

☐ Active participation in the treatment regimen

☐ Verbalization of reduced fear

Key interventions

• Assess the patient's and family members' verbal and nonverbal expressions of fear about the effects of hyperemesis gravidarum. Encourage open expression of feelings.

• Encourage open communication among the patient, family, and health care team.

• Provide accurate information in response to questions from the patient and family members.

• Help the patient and family assess previously successful methods of coping with fears. Encourage them to use these healthy coping methods.

• Teach the patient and family about the treatment regimen, and help them develop a plan to carry it out.

Multifetal pregnancy

Intrauterine pregnancy with more than one viable fetus.

NURSING DIAGNOSIS

Ineffective individual and family coping related to the increased physiologic and therapeutic demands imposed by multifetal pregnancy

DESIRED PATIENT OUTCOME

The patient and family will manage stress effectively and adapt to the demands of multifetal pregnancy

Outcome measurement criteria

☐ Correct identification of the increased physiologic and therapeutic demands of multifetal pregnancy

☐ Compliance with the therapeutic regimen

☐ Accurate verbalization of risk factors associated with multifetal pregnancy

☐ Accurate verbalization of signs of complications during pregnancy

☐ Use of effective coping techniques

Key interventions

• Assess the patient's and family's knowledge about the physiologic effects of multifetal pregnancy. Teach them about the physiologic demands of single-fetus pregnancy and the increased demands of multifetal pregnancy.

- Encourage adequate diet, rest, and exercise. Teach about the need for increased weight gain. Explain signs and symptoms of anemia during pregnancy and reinforce the need for vitamins and iron.

- Reinforce the need for antepartal visits with a health care professional every 2 weeks during the second trimester and weekly thereafter.

- Describe required laboratory and diagnostic tests.

- Explain the increased risk of complications during multifetal pregnancy. Teach the patient to recognize signs of such complications as preterm labor, pregnancy-induced hypertension, placenta previa, and abruptio placentae.

- Instruct the patient to monitor herself to detect contractions, absence of fetal movement, and clear or bloody vaginal discharge.

- Encourage the patient and her partner to alter their sexual practices during the third trimester to avoid orgasm, which increases the risk of uterine contractions.

- Help the patient and family understand and comply with the therapeutic regimen required for any complication of pregnancy.

- Teach about prescribed medications, including their administration schedule, benefits, and adverse effects.

- Reassure the patient that restrictions imposed by the pregnancy are transient and will not pose problems after the delivery.

- Help the patient and family maintain open communication and discuss their feelings about the effects of this pregnancy.

- Help them identify previously effective coping techniques. Support their use of safe, effective coping techniques and offer alternatives as needed.

NURSING DIAGNOSIS

Parental role conflict related to uncertainty about the ability to care for more than one infant

DESIRED PATIENT OUTCOME

The patient and family will successfully resolve concerns about their ability to care for multiple infants

Outcome measurement criteria

☐ Verbalization of specific concerns related to caring for multiple infants

☐ Participation in planning for care of infants

☐ Verbalization of realistic expectations about the ability to care for infants

☐ Demonstration of appropriate parental attachment

☐ Use of resources for additional support and help in caring for infants

☐ Verbalization of confidence about the ability to care for infants

Key interventions

• Help the patient and family discuss their concerns about the multifetal pregnancy. Encourage open communication among family members and health care professionals.

• Listen attentively to specific patient and family concerns and evaluate them carefully. Provide accurate information and correct misconceptions as needed.

• Help the patient and family plan for anticipated events associated with multiple birth. Encourage planning for mobilization of support from the family, community, church, and other support groups.

- Encourage evaluation of personal responsibilities and exploration of ways to integrate infant care successfully into the family's lifestyle.

- Help the patient and family establish realistic self-expectations related to infant care, depending on the infants' status at birth. Encourage family members to communicate with one another and with health care professionals about their desired level of participation in care.

- Assess the family's support systems. Refer to local and national organizations for information about coping with multiple births.

- Encourage the parents to plan time to meet their needs as a couple by regularly spending time together without their children.

Placenta previa

Abnormal placental implantation in the lower uterine segment so that the placenta marginally, partially, or completely occludes the cervical os.

NURSING DIAGNOSIS

Fear related to the effects of placenta previa on the pregnancy

DESIRED PATIENT OUTCOME

The patient will cope effectively with her fears about placenta previa and will participate in the plan of care

Outcome measurement criteria

- ☐ Verbalization of concerns about the maternal and fetal effects of placenta previa
- ☐ Verbalization of accurate understanding of the therapeutic regimen
- ☐ Participation in self-care to cope with fears
- ☐ Proper performance of self-monitoring for signs of fetal well-being and complications
- ☐ Report of reduced fear

Key interventions

- Encourage the patient to express feelings and concerns about placenta previa. Provide accurate information about its potential effects on maternal and fetal well-being.
- Teach about the therapeutic regimen, including the administration, benefits, and adverse effects of prescribed medications.

- Teach the patient how to monitor herself for signs and symptoms of pregnancy complications, such as abruptio placentae and preterm labor. Also teach her how to monitor for contractions and fetal movements; reassure her that fetal movements typically indicate fetal well-being.

- Tell the patient to notify a health care professional immediately if bleeding, cramping, or cessation of fetal movement occurs.

- Help the patient prepare for cesarean delivery. Explain the procedure and its implications for postpartal recovery.

- Reassess the patient's tolerance of fears at regular intervals.

NURSING DIAGNOSIS
Diversional activity deficit related to imposed bed rest secondary to placenta previa

DESIRED PATIENT OUTCOME
The patient will accept activity limitations and will engage in safe diversional activities

Outcome measurement criteria
- ☐ Verbalization of accurate understanding of the need to limit activity during pregnancy
- ☐ Verbalization of feelings about imposed activity limitations
- ☐ Correct identification of safe activities
- ☐ Involvement in safe activities and avoidance of unsafe activities
- ☐ Compliance with prescribed bed rest

Key interventions

- Explain the rationale for activity limitations.

- Encourage the patient and family members to discuss their feelings about activity limitations.

- Discuss various safe activities that the patient can perform within her activity limitations.

- Help the patient explore preferred or new safe activities, such as watching television or videotapes; listening to music or books on tape; reading; writing; doing needle-work; bird-watching; playing card, word, board, or video games; and talking with visitors.

- Help the patient develop a plan for coping with activity limitations when performing activities of daily living; for instance, folding clothes or preparing shopping lists while resting.

- Recommend periodic "changes of scenery" to avoid boredom. For example, the patient can rest on a couch or bed in different rooms at different times.

- Encourage mobilization of family and community support. Refer to community resources as needed.

NURSING DIAGNOSIS

Altered peripheral tissue perfusion related to excessive blood loss caused by placenta previa

DESIRED PATIENT OUTCOME

The patient will maintain adequate tissue perfusion to support maternal and fetal life

Outcome measurement criteria

☐ Vital signs within normal limits

☐ Urine output greater than 30 ml/hour

☐ Skin color within normal limits

☐ Normal capillary refill time

☐ Peripheral pulses present and equal

☐ Absence of lethargy or loss of consciousness

☐ Fluid intake that approximately equals output

☐ Fetal heart rate with reassuring pattern

Key interventions

- Assess vital signs frequently. Be alert for signs of hypovolemic shock, such as rapid, thready pulse; widening pulse pressure; and tachycardia.

- Use a continuous external fetal monitor to document fetal heart rate if the fetus is viable. Observe monitor tracings for signs of fetal well-being or distress. Document findings and notify the health care professional if nonreassuring patterns occur. If fetal mortality is inevitable, remove the external fetal monitor.

- Assess urine output frequently. Monitor and document urine volume and characteristics.

- Assess skin for diaphoresis, coolness, and color changes, such as pallor and nail bed cyanosis. Document findings.

- Assess and document the presence and strength of peripheral pulses.

- Assess and document level of consciousness.

- Document blood loss by recording the amount and character of loss over a specified period.

- Administer prescribed I.V. replacement fluids or blood products.

- Help prepare the patient for surgery if required. Place the patient in a lateral position and administer oxygen by face mask as prescribed.

Pregnancy-induced hypertension

Hypertensive disorder of pregnancy that includes preeclampsia and eclampsia and is characterized by a classic triad of symptoms: hypertension, edema, and proteinuria.

NURSING DIAGNOSIS

Ineffective management of therapeutic regimen related to lack of knowledge about pregnancy-induced hypertension (PIH) and the complexity of its treatment

DESIRED PATIENT OUTCOME

The patient will manage the therapeutic regimen for PIH effectively

Outcome measurement criteria

☐ Correct identification of self-monitoring techniques

☐ Use of effective self-monitoring techniques

☐ Accurate verbalization of the potential maternal and fetal effects of PIH

☐ Accurate verbalization of signs and symptoms of complications of PIH

☐ Correct identification of medications and other treatments for PIH

☐ Effective self-monitoring and use of medications and other treatments

☐ Absence of complications related to inability to manage the therapeutic regimen

Key interventions

- Assess the patient's knowledge of potential maternal and fetal risks of PIH. Explain these risks as the patient indicates a readiness to learn.

- Stress the importance of strict compliance with the prescribed therapeutic regimen to reduce the risk of complications. Teach the patient how to weigh herself daily, monitor blood pressure, assess for proteinuria, measure urine output, monitor fetal activity, assess for contractions, and limit sodium intake. Encourage frequent rest periods.

- Tell the patient to report promptly a weight gain of more than 1 lb (0.4 kg) per week, increasing edema, frequent headaches, vision disturbances, malaise, nausea, vomiting, increased blood pressure, decreased urine output, proteinuria of +2 or greater, contractions that occur before term, and decreased fetal movement.

- Teach the patient about prescribed and over-the-counter medications, including their safe dosage, benefits, adverse effects, and signs of toxicity.

- Stress the importance of attending all prenatal appointments and keeping a log of self-assessment information to share with the health care professional.

- Teach the patient about prescribed fetal assessment techniques.

- Verify the patient's understanding of all information provided; clarify misconceptions as needed. Acknowledge efforts toward self-care.

NURSING DIAGNOSIS

Diversional activity deficit related to imposed bed rest secondary to PIH

DESIRED PATIENT OUTCOME

The patient will accept activity limitations and will engage in safe diversional activities

Outcome measurement criteria

☐ Verbalization of accurate understanding of the need to limit activity during pregnancy

☐ Verbalization of feelings about imposed activity limitations

☐ Correct identification of safe activities

☐ Involvement in safe activities and avoidance of unsafe activities

☐ Compliance with prescribed bed rest

Key interventions

• Explain the rationale for activity limitations.

• Encourage the patient and family members to discuss their feelings about activity limitations.

• Discuss various safe activities that the patient can perform within her activity limitations.

• Help the patient explore preferred or new safe activities, such as watching television or videotapes; listening to music or books on tape; reading; writing; doing needlework; bird-watching; playing card, word, board, or video games; and talking with visitors.

• Help the patient develop a plan for coping with activity limitations when performing activities of daily living; for instance, folding clothes or preparing shopping lists while resting.

• Recommend periodic "changes of scenery" to avoid boredom. For example, the patient can rest on a couch or bed in different rooms at different times.

• Encourage mobilization of family and community support. Refer to community resources as needed.

NURSING DIAGNOSIS

High risk for injury (maternal and fetal) related to the effects of preeclampsia or its treatment

DESIRED PATIENT OUTCOME

The patient and fetus will remain free from injury during pregnancy

Outcome measurement criteria

☐ Absence of eclamptic seizures

☐ Respiratory rate greater than 12 breaths/minute

☐ Urine output greater than 30 ml/hour

☐ Absence of uteroplacental insufficiency

☐ Absence of preterm delivery

☐ Absence of abruptio placentae

Key interventions

• Administer medications and I.V. fluids as prescribed.

• Explain the plan of care to the patient and family members and provide reassurance as needed.

• Maintain a calm, quiet environment to decrease central nervous system stimulation. Place the patient in a lateral recumbent position and take seizure precautions at the bedside.

• Monitor and document blood pressure frequently. Notify the health care professional if it continues to increase.

• Assess and document deep tendon reflexes. Observe for absent or depressed reflexes.

• Closely assess the patient's respiratory pattern.

• Measure and record urine output hourly. Notify the health care professional if output falls below 30 ml/hour.

- Perform continuous external fetal monitoring. Document reassuring and nonreassuring patterns; report nonreassuring patterns. Change the patient's position as needed.

- Assess for signs of preterm labor, eclampsia, and abruptio placentae. Observe for contractions; increased blood pressure, edema, and proteinuria; and bleeding.

Premature rupture of membranes

Spontaneous rupture of amniotic membranes before term pregnancy and after the age of fetal viability.

NURSING DIAGNOSIS
High risk for infection related to premature rupture of membranes (PROM)

DESIRED PATIENT OUTCOME
The patient will remain free of uterine or fetal infection for the duration of pregnancy

Outcome measurement criteria
☐ Oral temperature at or below 99.0° F (37° C)

☐ White blood cell (WBC) count within normal limits

☐ Absence of uterine tenderness on palpation

☐ Absence of foul-smelling or excessive vaginal discharge

☐ Clear to white vaginal discharge

☐ Verbalization and demonstration of effective measures to prevent infection

☐ Verbalization and demonstration of effective self-monitoring techniques for signs of infection

☐ Verbalization of accurate knowledge about medication use

☐ Correct identification of reportable symptoms

☐ Verbalization of the correct procedure to follow to report signs and symptoms of infection

Key interventions

- Assess oral temperature every 4 to 6 hours; report temperature over 99.0° F (37.2° C).

- Obtain WBC count as prescribed; report increased values.

- Assess the patient's response to uterine palpation. Be alert for pain on palpation.

- Assess the quantity, odor, and appearance of vaginal drainage. Document and report any changes.

- Limit the patient's activity to bed rest with bathroom privileges.

- Avoid performing vaginal examinations.

- Explain the significance of and procedures for self-monitoring of temperature, uterine tenderness, and vaginal discharge. Instruct the patient to report any abnormal signs and symptoms.

- Instruct the patient to avoid intercourse, douches, and tampons. Teach appropriate hygiene measures to use after elimination.

- Teach the patient the purpose, dosage, benefits, and adverse effects of prescribed medications.

Nursing Diagnosis

Altered family processes related to situational crisis secondary to PROM

DESIRED PATIENT OUTCOME

The patient and family will adapt positively to changes in family processes

Outcome measurement criteria

☐ Open verbalization of feelings about family situation

☐ Verbalization of understanding that changes in family processes are temporary and result from the situation

☐ Active participation in plans for solving family problems resulting from the situation

☐ Active participation in problem resolution within imposed activity limitations

Key interventions

• Help the patient examine the situation's impact on family processes, including financial implications, changes in role expectations, and social limitations.

• Encourage expression of feelings about the effect of this situation on family processes. Promote open communication among family members.

• Encourage the family to develop a plan for adapting to changes in financial situation, role expectations, and social interactions as needed.

• Help the patient and family recognize that the effects of this situation on family processes are temporary.

• Help the patient and family explore resources for assistance with adaptation, such as community organizations, other family members, and friends.

• Provide information about and referrals to social services and other resources for assistance with homemaker activities, meal preparation, and financial management.

• Help the family plan to include the patient in problem solving within the limitations of her imposed restrictions.

• Encourage maintenance of open communication.

NURSING DIAGNOSIS

Fear related to unknown pregnancy outcome

DESIRED PATIENT OUTCOME

The patient will report confidence in her ability to cope with unknown pregnancy outcome

Outcome measurement criteria

☐ Verbalization of fears or concerns about the pregnancy outcome

☐ Verbalization of absence of self-blame

☐ Calm, relaxed appearance and verbalization that fears are reduced

☐ Use of appropriate resources to decrease fear

Key interventions

• Assess the patient's level of fear about the pregnancy outcome. Encourage discussion of fears or concerns.

• Acknowledge the patient's fears and concerns. Correct misinformation as needed.

• Reassure the patient that her emotional lability is normal, and encourage her to acknowledge and express all emotions.

• Reinforce the unavoidability of PROM; encourage the patient to avoid blaming herself.

• Assist the patient to identify previously successful coping mechanisms. Encourage her to use healthy coping mechanisms and avoid unhealthy ones.

• Provide accurate information about the prognosis as the patient desires. Provide written information about managing PROM as needed and desired by the patient.

• Help the patient compile a list of techniques, such as deep-breathing and relaxation exercises, to help her control anxiety. Assist in planning measures to decrease anxiety by using these techniques.

Preterm labor

Spontaneous onset of labor after the age of fetal viability but before term gestation.

NURSING DIAGNOSIS

Fear related to the unknown effects of preterm labor on the pregnancy outcome

DESIRED PATIENT OUTCOME

The patient and family will manage fear effectively and demonstrate relaxation

Outcome measurement criteria

☐ Verbalization of specific concerns about the pregnancy outcome

☐ Verbalization of effective coping mechanisms

☐ Exploration of options for coping with specific fears

☐ Demonstration of effective problem-solving skills

☐ Report of reduced fear

Key interventions

• Establish a rapport with the patient and family. Encourage open expression of general and specific concerns.

• Help the patient and family obtain accurate information about the potential effects of preterm labor as they desire.

• Promote exploration of previously successful techniques for coping with stress. Reinforce positive coping techniques.

- Encourage the patient and family to be involved in problem solving about the pregnancy. Praise their efforts toward making decisions.

- Refer the patient and family to community resources, counselors, or support groups as needed.

NURSING DIAGNOSIS

Ineffective management of therapeutic regimen related to lack of knowledge about and complexity of therapy for preterm labor

DESIRED PATIENT OUTCOME

The patient will effectively manage the therapeutic regimen

Outcome measurement criteria

☐ Correct identification of the risks of preterm labor

☐ Correct identification of signs of preterm labor

☐ Demonstration of effective self-monitoring techniques

☐ Verbalization of accurate knowledge about pharmacologic treatment for preterm labor

☐ Verbalization of the need for increased rest or complete bed rest during pregnancy

☐ Compliance with the prescribed self-monitoring, pharmacologic, and activity regimens

☐ Verbalization of the proper procedure to follow to report recurrence of preterm labor

☐ Absence of complications of preterm labor

Key interventions

- Assess the patient's knowledge of the risks of preterm labor; provide information as needed. Explain that each day without preterm labor increases the fetus's likelihood of survival.

- Discuss the signs of preterm labor, especially uterine contractions. Teach the patient how to monitor for uterine activity and fetal activity, using a home uterine activity monitor if indicated.

- Reinforce the need for increased rest to help decrease uterine activity.

- Teach about pharmacologic management of preterm labor. Administer I.V. medications and fluids as prescribed in the hospital. Teach appropriate self-administration by the oral or subcutaneous route for home use, as prescribed. Explain the benefits, risks, and adverse effects of all prescribed medications.

- Instruct the patient to report increased uterine activity promptly. Explain that treatment is more likely to be effective when started within 72 hours of labor onset.

- Verify the patient's understanding of the regimen. Provide written information to reinforce instructions.

- Assess the patient's ability to manage the therapeutic regimen during follow-up visits.

NURSING DIAGNOSIS

Diversional activity deficit related to imposed bed rest secondary to preterm labor

DESIRED PATIENT OUTCOME

The patient will accept activity limitations and will engage in safe diversional activities

Outcome measurement criteria

☐ Verbalization of accurate understanding of the need to limit activity during pregnancy

☐ Verbalization of feelings about imposed activity limitations

☐ Correct identification of safe activities

☐ Involvement in safe activities and avoidance of unsafe activities

☐ Compliance with prescribed bed rest

Key interventions

• Explain the rationale for activity limitations.

• Encourage the patient and family members to discuss their feelings about activity limitations.

• Discuss various safe activities that the patient can perform within her activity limitations.

• Help the patient explore preferred or new safe activities, such as watching television or videotapes; listening to music or books on tape; reading; writing; doing needlework; bird-watching; playing card, word, board, or video games; and talking with visitors.

• Help the patient develop a plan for coping with activity limitations when performing activities of daily living; for instance, folding clothes or preparing shopping lists while resting.

• Recommend periodic "changes of scenery" to avoid boredom. For example, the patient can rest on a couch or bed in different rooms at different times.

• Encourage mobilization of family and community support. Refer to community resources as needed.

NURSING DIAGNOSIS

Constipation related to decreased GI activity caused by imposed bed rest and the adverse effects of tocolytics

DESIRED PATIENT OUTCOME

The patient will maintain normal bowel function throughout pregnancy

Outcome measurement criteria

☐ Correct identification and effective use of dietary and physical measures to promote GI motility

☐ Verbalization of accurate understanding of prescribed drug to promote bowel elimination

☐ Absence of hard, dry stools

☐ Maintenance of normal bowel elimination pattern

Key interventions

• Assess the patient's knowledge of dietary practices to promote bowel elimination. Help her review and evaluate a typical 24-hour intake.

• Teach the patient to increase her fiber and fluid intake and to perform limited leg exercises in bed.

• Describe proper positioning to promote bowel elimination (using a footstool in front of the toilet to elevate the feet).

• Teach the patient about the use of stool softeners. Encourage her to consult a health care professional before using any medications.

• Reassess dietary practices and bowel elimination at follow-up visits.

Sexually transmitted diseases

Infections by organisms spread predominantly or exclusively through sexual contact.

NURSING DIAGNOSIS

Ineffective management of therapeutic regimen related to lack of knowledge about disease transmission, treatment, and prevention

DESIRED PATIENT OUTCOME

The patient will manage her therapeutic regimen appropriately and will gain accurate knowledge of transmission, treatment, and prevention of sexually transmitted diseases (STDs)

Outcome measurement criteria

☐ Accurate description of the prescribed treatment regimen

☐ Correct identification of transmission routes and ways to prevent transmission

☐ Compliance with the prescribed treatment regimen

☐ Verbalization and use of practices to avoid reinfection of self or infection of fetus or partner

Key interventions

• Assess the patient's knowledge of the prescribed treatment regimen. Teach about the appropriate use, benefits, and adverse effects of medications and other treatment measures. Reinforce the need to complete the entire course of treatment.

- Advise the patient to refrain from intercourse if perineal irritation or inflammation occurs.

- Encourage the patient to refrain from intercourse until her partner receives treatment, if indicated. Explain that she could become reinfected after successful treatment if her partner remains untreated.

- Assess the patient's knowledge about her infection and the effects of STDs in general. Using language appropriate to the patient's ability to understand, provide accurate information and clarify misconceptions.

- Assess the patient's knowledge about preventing STD transmission. Discuss specific high-risk practices and prevention techniques.

- Reinforce the need to limit the number of sexual partners (preferably to one), use condoms and spermicide with a new partner or any partner who has multiple sexual contacts, inspect herself and her partner for lesions or discharge, and abstain from intercourse if oral or genital lesions or an unusual discharge appears.

- Encourage the patient to return for scheduled follow-up visits with health care professionals and seek accurate answers to further questions from appropriate sources.

NURSING DIAGNOSIS

Personal identity disturbance related to the impact of an STD

DESIRED PATIENT OUTCOME

The patient will use effective coping mechanisms and will express self-acceptance

Outcome measurement criteria
☐ Expression of acceptance of the diagnosis

☐ Absence of statements indicating negative self-perception related to the STD

☐ Verbalization of effective plans to avoid future STD infection

Key interventions

• Promote open communication in a nonjudgmental atmosphere.

• Assess the patient's self-concept. Encourage her to express her feelings about the STD; be alert for indications of denial.

• Encourage the patient in denial to express general fears and concerns. Gradually focus the conversation on concerns specific to the STD.

• Be alert for statements that indicate negative self-concept. Explore reasons for negative self-concept and provide accurate, nonjudgmental information in response to questions. Clarify misconceptions as needed.

• Help the patient develop a plan to avoid reinfection or transmission of STDs. Acknowledge her accurate understanding of disease control and prevention. Correct any misconceptions as needed.

NURSING DIAGNOSIS

Altered family processes related to the effects of the STD on family relationships

DESIRED PATIENT OUTCOME

The patient and family will adapt successfully to stressors and will resume effective functioning

Outcome measurement criteria

☐ Safe, effective expression of feelings and concerns

☐ Participation in a plan of care to decrease the risk of reinfection

☐ Report of continuation of supportive roles within the family

☐ Use of external resources as needed

Key interventions

- Help the patient and family evaluate the effects of the STD. Provide a safe environment for expression of feelings. Be alert for indications of additional family stressors.

- Teach effective communication skills in a safe, therapeutic manner. Stress the importance of open communication to problem solving.

- Recognize previously effective problem-solving skills. Encourage both partners to participate in developing a plan to cope effectively with stressors.

- Provide information about STD treatment, transmission prevention, and potential for reinfection.

- Refer the patient and family to community agencies, counseling services, clergy, and other sources of support as needed.

Spontaneous abortion

Naturally occurring expulsion of the fetus before the age of viability.

NURSING DIAGNOSIS

High risk for dysfunctional grieving related to pregnancy loss

DESIRED PATIENT OUTCOME

The patient and family will progress through the stages of grief and express hope for future pregnancies

Outcome measurement criteria

- ☐ Verbalization of the effect of this loss on self and family
- ☐ Verbalization of accurate knowledge about spontaneous abortion and its effect on future pregnancies
- ☐ Performance of appropriate self-care
- ☐ Use of external supports as needed

Key interventions

- Establish a therapeutic relationship with the patient and family and validate the spontaneous abortion as a real loss. When they are ready, discuss the stages of grief.
- Encourage the patient and family to discuss their feelings about the effects of the loss.
- Encourage the patient and family to accept and recognize differences in individual and cultural responses to grief and to recognize the need for individual progress through the stages of grief.

- Provide accurate information about the incidence and causes of spontaneous abortion and about its effect on future pregnancies.

- Reassure the patient and family that ambivalence is normal early in pregnancy and does not cause spontaneous abortion.

- Teach the patient appropriate self-care measures: avoidance of pregnancy for the next 3 months; avoidance of douches, tampons, and intercourse until bleeding has stopped; RhoGAM administration if the patient is Rh negative; and correct use of prescribed medications. Encourage her to rest frequently to promote emotional and physical recovery.

- Reassure the patient and family that some emotional lability is normal after spontaneous abortion.

- Provide information about support groups, counselors, clergy, and telephone support lines. Encourage the use of these or other resources if depression occurs or grief does not resolve.

NURSING DIAGNOSIS

High risk for fluid volume deficit related to excessive blood loss secondary to spontaneous abortion

DESIRED PATIENT OUTCOME

The patient will demonstrate no signs or symptoms of fluid volume deficit

Outcome measurement criteria

☐ Absence of signs of dehydration
☐ Vital signs within normal limits
☐ Laboratory test results within normal limits

Key interventions

- Monitor and document vital signs, weight, skin turgor, mucous membrane color and moisture, and capillary refill time.

- Monitor and record fluid intake and output. Teach the patient and family the rationale for this measure and instruct them to measure and document fluid intake and output at home.

- Monitor vaginal loss of blood by documenting its quantity, appearance, and odor. Calculate the number of pads used and the approximate percentage of pad soaked in a time period.

- Teach the patient to promptly report heavy, bright red, or increased bleeding.

- Monitor laboratory test results as indicated. Note and report any significant decrease in hemoglobin and hematocrit values.

- Administer I.V. fluids as prescribed.

Substance abuse during pregnancy

Use of tobacco, alcohol, or psychoactive substances by a pregnant woman.

NURSING DIAGNOSIS

High risk for ineffective management of therapeutic regimen related to addiction or dependence, inconsistent participation in prenatal care, and lack of knowledge of the potentially harmful effects of substance abuse

DESIRED PATIENT OUTCOME

The patient will manage her prenatal care regimen effectively, will control substance abuse, and will receive consistent prenatal care

Outcome measurement criteria

☐ Attendance at all scheduled prenatal visits

☐ Accurate identification of dietary needs during pregnancy

☐ Appropriate weight gain from an adequate diet

☐ Verbalization of maternal and fetal risks of substance abuse

☐ Accurate identification of signs and symptoms of preterm labor and abruptio placentae

☐ Verbalization of accurate understanding of the prescribed medication regimen

☐ Participation in an appropriate drug rehabilitation program

Key interventions

- Teach the patient the importance of regular monitoring at prenatal visits, and strongly encourage her to receive all available prenatal care.

- Assess the patient's ability to attend scheduled prenatal visits. Help her arrange for transportation or other assistance if needed.

- Teach the patient about desired weight gain during pregnancy, and document her weight changes at each prenatal visit.

- Assess the patient's ability to obtain sufficient nutritious food. If needed, refer her to community resources or social services, such as the Special Supplemental Food Program for Women, Infants, and Children (WIC).

- Teach the patient about her prescribed medications, including their appropriate use, correct dosage, benefits, and adverse effects.

- Discuss the potential fetal effects of the substance the patient abuses. Describe specific risks to the fetus, and encourage the patient to view her pregnancy as a motivation to overcome her addiction.

- Support any efforts the patient makes to deal with the addiction, such as enrolling in a rehabilitation program, participating in a support group, or controlling her drug use.

- Give the patient information about drug treatment programs, refer her for counseling, and identify appropriate support groups.

- Explain the signs and symptoms of preterm labor and abruptio placentae; encourage the patient to notify her health care professional promptly if they occur.

NURSING DIAGNOSIS

High risk for ineffective individual coping related to inability to manage stress without the use of drugs

DESIRED PATIENT OUTCOME

The patient will manage the stresses of daily life appropriately while abstaining from the abuse of drugs

Outcome measurement criteria

☐ Verbalization of a plan for dealing with stress constructively

☐ Demonstration of learned techniques for coping with stress without the use of drugs

☐ Verbalization of the need for continued abstinence from drugs

☐ Report of use of new coping techniques and abstinence from drugs

Key interventions

• Help the patient establish goals for coping with pregnancy and substance abuse.

• Encourage the patient to identify successful coping techniques that she used in stressful situations in the past. Also ask her to discuss her motivation to succeed in coping with these situations. Help her develop a plan for using similar techniques to cope with daily life without the use of drugs.

• Help the patient examine stressors in her life, such as financial concerns, emotional problems, an unsupportive family, or problems with other children. As appropriate, refer her to community resources for assistance in meeting her needs.

- Assist the patient to explore effective coping techniques. Verbally rehearse or role-play stressful situations with the patient. Encourage her to explore new, positive ways to cope with stress.

- Encourage the patient's participation in support groups and provide referrals as needed.

- Assess the patient's understanding of the need to abstain from drug use during pregnancy. Praise appropriate understanding.

- Reassess the patient's coping techniques on follow-up visits.

TORCH infections

Infections caused by organisms that may cross the placental barrier and cause serious fetal damage. The acronym TORCH refers to toxoplasmosis, other infections (including syphilis, hepatitis B virus, and group B beta-hemolytic streptococcus), rubella, and cytomegalovirus and herpes simplex infections.

NURSING DIAGNOSIS

Anticipatory grieving related to the infection's potential effects on the fetus

DESIRED PATIENT OUTCOME

The patient and family will acknowledge grief associated with the infection and will become actively involved in the plan of care

Outcome measurement criteria

- ☐ Participation in decision making related to care of the mother and fetus
- ☐ Use of external support as needed
- ☐ Resolution of grief

Key interventions

- Promote open communication among family members and health care professionals. Provide information about grieving and help family members recognize behaviors associated with the stages of grief.

- Encourage the patient and family to accept and recognize differences in individual and cultural responses to grief. Encourage them to recognize that each person progresses through grief at his or her individual pace.

- Refer the patient and family to community agencies, support groups, clergy, or counselors as needed.
- Encourage the patient and family to be involved in making decisions about managing the pregnancy. Answer questions honestly and correct misconceptions as needed.
- Support the patient's and family's decision-making efforts and commend effective coping mechanisms.

NURSING DIAGNOSIS

Ineffective management of therapeutic regimen related to inadequate knowledge of the cause, treatment, prevention, and risks associated with the infection

DESIRED PATIENT OUTCOME

The patient will manage the therapeutic regimen effectively and will demonstrate accurate knowledge of the infection's implications

Outcome measurement criteria

☐ Verbalization of accurate knowledge about the infection's cause

☐ Correct identification of personal and fetal risks associated with the infection

☐ Verbalization of effective ways to prevent infection transmission

☐ Accurate description of the required therapeutic regimen

☐ Compliance with the therapeutic regimen

Key interventions

- Assess the patient's knowledge of the infection. Provide accurate information appropriate to the patient's readiness to learn and ability to understand. Clarify misconceptions as needed.

- Teach the patient about required diagnostic tests. Help her obtain accurate information about test results.

- Teach the patient about the cause of the infection and ways the organism is transmitted. Provide accurate information about potential maternal and fetal effects of the infection.

- Help the patient fully understand the required treatment regimen. Teach about prescribed medication, treatments, and laboratory and diagnostic tests.

- Instruct the patient about methods to prevent disease transmission to the fetus and others.

- Refer the patient to support groups, community agencies, and additional information sources as needed.

NURSING DIAGNOSIS

High risk for infection (fetal) related to exposure to organisms from the pregnant patient

DESIRED PATIENT OUTCOME

The pregnant patient will take actions to prevent infection of her fetus

Outcome measurement criteria

☐ Correct identification of ways to prevent fetal infection

☐ Accurate verbalization of signs of fetal infection

☐ Use of techniques to avoid infection by the patient and her family

Key interventions

- Teach the patient and family about hand-washing and general hygiene techniques as ways to control infection transmission.

- Teach the patient to recognize the signs of membrane rupture. Advise her to notify a health care professional if spontaneous rupture of membranes occurs.

- Describe signs of fetal compromise, such as preterm labor, vaginal bleeding, and absence of fetal movement. Urge the patient to notify a health care professional immediately if these signs occur.

- For related information, see "Infections" in the Intrapartal Period section.

Trauma or battering during pregnancy

Physical injury to a pregnant woman caused by trauma or physical abuse.

NURSING DIAGNOSIS
Pain related to injuries secondary to trauma or battering

DESIRED PATIENT OUTCOME
The patient will experience decreased pain from injuries

Outcome measurement criteria
☐ Absence of signs of pain
☐ Verbalization of appropriate pharmacologic and non-pharmacologic pain-relief methods
☐ Report of decreased pain

Key interventions
- Assess the patient's level of pain. Encourage her to communicate the need for assistance with pain relief.
- Teach the patient about prescribed drugs for pain control, including their safe dosage, benefits, and adverse effects.
- Teach the patient about various nonpharmacologic pain-relief methods, including relaxation, massage, ice packs, and heating pads. Provide nonpharmacologic pain control as the patient requests.
- Reassess the patient's pain regularly.

NURSING DIAGNOSIS

Fear related to the actual or perceived fetal effects of the maternal physical injury

DESIRED PATIENT OUTCOME

The patient will express decreased fear about the effects of her injuries on the fetus

Outcome measurement criteria

☐ Verbalization of specific concerns about the effects of injuries on the fetus

☐ Expression of accurate understanding of diagnostic tests performed to determine fetal well-being

Key interventions

• Encourage the patient to discuss concerns about the fetus's well-being. Maintain open communication.

• Teach the patient about the procedures involved in assessing fetal well-being.

• Provide accurate information about fetal status. Use assessment techniques that provide audible and visual reassurance of fetal well-being, such as Doppler ultrasonography and ultrasonography.

• Reassess fetal status as ordered and reassure the patient as needed.

NURSING DIAGNOSIS

High risk for injury (fetal) related to preterm labor or abruptio placentae secondary to physical injuries from or surgical intervention for trauma or battering

DESIRED PATIENT OUTCOME

The fetus will remain free from injury caused by preterm labor or abruptio placentae

Outcome measurement criteria

☐ Absence of persistent uterine contractions

☐ Absence of bloody vaginal discharge

☐ Absence of rigid maternal abdomen

☐ Reassuring fetal heart rate (FHR) pattern

Key interventions

- Teach the patient to report unusual sensations in the abdomen, vagina, back, or shoulders; these sensations may indicate abruptio placentae.

- Assess the patient's abdomen for rigidity or increasing firmness; report rigidity or increasing firmness to the health care professional.

- Assess and document the amount, color, consistency, and odor of vaginal drainage. Notify the health care professional of any vaginal discharge.

- Maintain the patient in a lateral recumbent position to promote uteroplacental circulation.

- Assess FHR, noting reassuring and nonreassuring patterns. Notify the health care professional if nonreassuring patterns occur.

NURSING DIAGNOSIS

Hopelessness related to prolonged exposure to violence

DESIRED PATIENT OUTCOME

The patient will report a feeling of control over her life and hope for her future

Outcome measurement criteria

☐ Acknowledgment of self-worth and absence of self-blame

☐ Verbalization of personal strengths

☐ Identification of various resources for assistance

☐ Report of appropriate plans for managing immediate needs

Key interventions

- Encourage the patient to talk about the abuse. Use active listening techniques, and convey concern and empathy.

- Discuss the typical cycle of domestic violence, and encourage the patient to view herself as a victim. Stress that she deserves respect and does not deserve to be victimized.

- Help the patient examine her personal strengths and coping skills. Focus on and reinforce coping techniques that were successful in the past.

- Assess the patient's knowledge of available resources, such as shelters, support groups, financial aid, and child care. Provide information as needed.

- Help the patient develop a plan for coping with immediate needs for protection, child care, and financial support. Refer her to social services as needed.

- Remain accepting of the patient even if she chooses to return to the abusive situation.

Urinary tract infection

Bacterial infection affecting the urethra (urethritis), urinary bladder (cystitis), or the renal pelvis (pyelonephritis).

NURSING DIAGNOSIS

Pain related to urinary tract infection (UTI)

DESIRED PATIENT OUTCOME

The patient will experience no pain on urination

Outcome measurement criteria

☐ Absence of signs of inflammation

☐ Report of absence of pain

☐ Verbalization of effective pain-relief measures

☐ Use of appropriate methods to relieve pain

Key interventions

- Assess for verbal and nonverbal indications of pain associated with UTI, including costovertebral angle tenderness, suprapubic pain, nausea, vomiting, back pain, and malaise.

- Administer I.V. fluids, analgesics, antibiotics, and other medications as prescribed. Teach the patient about the benefits, adverse effects, and appropriate use of each medication.

NURSING DIAGNOSIS

Ineffective management of therapeutic regimen related to insufficient knowledge of the cause, prevention, treatment, and risks of UTI

DESIRED PATIENT OUTCOME

The patient will manage the therapeutic regimen for UTI effectively

Outcome measurement criteria

☐ Correct identification of the cause, signs, and symptoms of UTI

☐ Verbalization of effective self-care techniques

☐ Use of appropriate self-care techniques to avoid reinfection

☐ Compliance with the prescribed pharmacologic regimen

☐ Accurate verbalization of the risks associated with untreated UTI during the antepartal and postpartal periods

Key interventions

• Describe the increased risk of UTI during the antepartal and postpartal periods caused by anatomic and physiologic changes in the woman's body.

• Teach the patient to recognize signs and symptoms of UTI, such as urinary frequency or urgency, dysuria, urinary hesitancy, enuresis, dribbling, hematuria, fever, flank pain, nausea, and vomiting. Advise her to avoid complications by seeking prompt treatment if these signs and symptoms occur.

• Teach the patient these measures to prevent UTIs from recurring: wiping from front to back after urinating or defecating, using only mild cleansers when bathing, avoiding perfumed soaps or perineal sprays, wearing cotton underclothes, sleeping without underclothes, avoiding tight-fitting clothing, keeping the perineum dry, frequently changing moist pads, voiding before and after intercourse, avoiding sexual practices that traumatize the urethral area, voiding frequently, maintaining adequate fluid intake (8 to 10 glasses of fluid per day), and seeking early treatment for symptoms of vaginitis.

- Instruct the patient how to use pharmacologic agents properly. Reinforce the importance of completing the course of prescribed medications and returning for a urine culture, if required.

- Explain that untreated UTI increases the risk of preterm labor, permanent renal damage, and generalized sepsis.

Vaginitis

Overgrowth of Candida albicans *or* Gardnerella vaginalis *that causes inflammation of the vaginal mucosa or vulva.*

NURSING DIAGNOSIS

Impaired tissue integrity related to pruritus, excoriation, and inflammation caused by vaginitis

DESIRED PATIENT OUTCOME

The patient will participate in self-care and will exhibit healing of damaged tissue

Outcome measurement criteria

☐ Correct identification of the cause, treatment, and risks of vaginitis

☐ Use of appropriate methods to decrease and prevent perineal tissue damage

☐ Absence of signs of perineal or vaginal tissue damage

☐ Report of physical comfort

Key interventions

• Assess the degree of damage to perineal tissue.

• Teach the patient about the appearance of healthy perineal tissue and help her evaluate the appearance of her perineum. Show her how to use a mirror for self-inspection, and encourage regular self-inspection.

• Describe causative organisms and explain that this condition results from overgrowth of normal flora. Explain how pregnancy increases the risk for such infections.

- Teach about prescribed medications, including their appropriate use, benefits, and adverse effects. Warn against using tampons when using a prescribed vaginal cream.

- Discuss these potential risks of untreated vaginitis during pregnancy and delivery: urinary tract infection, fetal infection during delivery, preterm labor, premature rupture of membranes, and postpartal endometriosis.

- Assess the patient's knowledge of ways to avoid reinfection and care for herself during the infection. As needed, instruct her to avoid scratching or rubbing irritated perineal skin. Also teach about urogenital hygiene measures: wearing only cotton underclothing, sleeping without underclothing after treatment is completed, avoiding tight-fitting clothing, increasing the intake of yogurt or acidophilus milk during *Candida* infections, avoiding intercourse during vaginal irritation, avoiding sexual practices that may irritate perineal tissue, and changing moist perineal pads frequently.

- Reinforce the need to complete the course of prescribed treatment and to notify a health care professional of infection recurrence or treatment ineffectiveness.

NURSING DIAGNOSIS

Altered sexuality patterns related to dyspareunia from vaginitis

DESIRED PATIENT OUTCOME

The patient and her partner will express satisfaction with altered sexual practices during acute illness

Outcome measurement criteria

☐ Verbalization of the need for altering sexual practices during acute illness

☐ Communication with partner about acceptable sexual practices

☐ Exploration of alternative methods of sexual expression

☐ Use of appropriate methods to obtain sexual satisfaction

Key interventions

- Establish a therapeutic relationship with the patient and her partner. Encourage open discussion of concerns and feelings related to the need to alter sexual practices during treatment of vaginitis.

- Assess or encourage the patient and partner to assess previous sexual practices to determine the need to avoid potentially damaging activities.

- Discuss safe, alternative means of sexual expression that the patient and partner might use during acute illness.

- Reassure the patient and partner that vaginitis is transient and that they should be able to resume their previous sexual activity when the infection is resolved.

- Decrease the risk of tissue trauma by encouraging the use of a water-soluble lubricant as needed when intercourse is resumed.

Abruptio placentae

Premature detachment of part or all of a normally implanted placenta.

NURSING DIAGNOSIS

Pain related to increased intrauterine pressure secondary to bleeding from abruptio placentae

DESIRED PATIENT OUTCOME

The patient will experience decreased pain

Outcome measurement criteria

☐ Absence of signs and symptoms of pain

☐ Verbalization of pain tolerance

Key interventions

- Assess the patient's response to her condition. Be alert for signs and symptoms of pain.

- Explain the source of the pain. Provide reassurance and comfort measures as needed.

- Reinforce the patient's understanding that the pain is temporary.

- Help the patient engage in diversional activities, such as controlled breathing.

- Administer pain medications as prescribed.

NURSING DIAGNOSIS

Altered fetal tissue perfusion related to decreased placental circulation secondary to abruptio placentae

DESIRED PATIENT OUTCOME

The patient will maintain sufficient placental circulation to sustain fetal life until delivery

Outcome measurement criteria

☐ Fetal heart rate (FHR) of 120 to 160 beats/minute

☐ Average short-term variability and long-term variability in FHR

☐ Absence of nonreassuring FHR patterns

☐ FHR acceleration with fetal movement

☐ Delivery of a viable infant

Key interventions

- Notify the appropriate health team members upon identification of abruptio placentae, and prepare for an emergency delivery.

- Monitor and document FHR continually; be alert for variability and nonreassuring patterns.

- Reposition the patient as necessary to promote circulation through remaining intact placental structures.

- Administer oxygen at 8 to 10 liters/minute through a tight face mask, as prescribed.

- Carry out orders to promote hastened delivery. Assist with preparation for cesarean delivery, as ordered.

NURSING DIAGNOSIS

High risk for fluid volume deficit related to excessive blood loss secondary to concealed or frank hemorrhage

DESIRED PATIENT OUTCOME

The patient will maintain adequate fluid volume and electrolyte balance

Outcome measurement criteria

☐ Blood pressure within normal range for the patient

☐ Absence of narrowed pulse pressure

☐ Pulse rate of 60 to 90 beats/minute

☐ Strong peripheral pulses

☐ Skin warm to touch with no mottling or cyanosis

☐ Absence of confusion and loss of consciousness

☐ Urine output greater than or equal to 30 ml/hour

☐ Electrolyte and blood component values within normal ranges

☐ Coagulation study results within normal ranges

☐ Hemodynamic monitoring values within normal ranges

Key interventions

• Assess and document vital signs frequently.

• Assess and document level of consciousness.

• Administer I.V. fluids, medications, and blood components, as prescribed.

• Assist with interpreting and reporting requested laboratory studies, such as hematocrit and hemoglobin and electrolyte levels.

• Assist with insertion of an internal monitoring device as required.

• Monitor and document fluid intake and output and the patient's hemodynamic status.

• Assess for signs and symptoms of a clotting disorder, such as epistaxis and bleeding from injection sites. Document and promptly report such findings.

NURSING DIAGNOSIS

Fear related to inadequate knowledge about treatment for abruptio placentae and the disorder's potential effects on maternal and fetal well-being

DESIRED PATIENT OUTCOME

The patient and family will express increased knowledge about treatment for abruptio placentae and will cope effectively with their fears about its potential effects

Outcome measurement criteria

☐ Verbalization of accurate understanding of the treatment regimen

☐ Acknowledgment of the need for treatment

☐ Acknowledgment and discussion of concerns

☐ Demonstration of appropriate range of affect

Key interventions

- Maintain a calm, professional demeanor at the patient's bedside and with family members.

- Assess the patient's and family's emotional reaction to the situation.

- Help the patient and family understand the need for treatment. Explain the rationale for all treatment measures.

- Keep the patient and family informed about maternal and fetal status throughout treatment.

- Encourage the patient and family to ask questions.

- Assist the patient and family to identify and draw on available resources (such as other family members, other health care professionals, counselors, and clergy) to promote discussion of feelings.

- For related information, see "Family adaptation to loss of an infant" in the Postpartal Period section.

Amniotic fluid embolism

A rare, life-threatening complication that occurs when an embolus of amniotic fluid is forced into maternal circulation and blocks an artery.

NURSING DIAGNOSIS

Inability to sustain spontaneous ventilation related to compromised cardiopulmonary status secondary to amniotic fluid embolism

DESIRED PATIENT OUTCOME

The patient will maintain adequate respiratory status to sustain maternal and fetal life

Outcome measurement criteria

☐ Respiratory rate of 12 to 20 breaths/minute

☐ Lungs clear during auscultation

☐ Absence of dyspnea, restlessness, or apprehension

☐ No accessory muscle use

☐ Ability to clear mucus and fluid from the respiratory tract

☐ Tidal volume within normal range

☐ Arterial blood gas (ABG) values within normal ranges

Key interventions

• Assess and document respiratory status frequently.

• Assess for indications of respiratory distress, including adventitious breath sounds, apprehension, restlessness, accessory muscle use, and pink, frothy sputum.

- Reposition the patient as necessary to ease ventilatory effort.
- Assess and document the patient's ability to clear the respiratory tract. Suction as necessary.
- Assist with evaluation of tidal volume and ABG values as indicated.
- Administer medications as prescribed.
- Assist with intubation as indicated.
- Initiate or assist with resuscitative efforts as indicated.

NURSING DIAGNOSIS

Altered placental and peripheral tissue perfusion related to compromised cardiovascular status secondary to amniotic fluid embolism

DESIRED PATIENT OUTCOME

The patient will maintain adequate circulating blood volume to sustain maternal and fetal life

Outcome measurement criteria

☐ Blood pressure within normal range for the patient

☐ Absence of narrowing pulse pressure

☐ Maternal pulse rate between 60 and 90 beats/minute

☐ No loss of consciousness

☐ Absence of cardiac arrhythmias

☐ Urine output greater than or equal to 30 ml/hour

☐ Palpable peripheral pulses

☐ Fetal heart rate (FHR) between 120 and 160 beats/minute

☐ Absence of nonreassuring FHR pattern

Key interventions

- Assess and document maternal vital signs frequently.
- Use an electronic fetal monitoring device to frequently assess and document FHR patterns.
- Use an electronic monitoring device to frequently assess and document maternal cardiac rhythms.
- Assess the patient's level of consciousness.
- Insert an indwelling bladder catheter as ordered. Assess and document the quantity and character of urine output.
- Assess and document peripheral pulses.
- Administer emergency or supportive medications as prescribed.
- Initiate or assist with resuscitative efforts as indicated.

NURSING DIAGNOSIS

Fear related to inadequate knowledge about treatment and the potential effects of amniotic fluid embolism on maternal and fetal well-being

DESIRED PATIENT OUTCOME

The patient and family will express increased knowledge about treatment for amniotic fluid embolism and will cope effectively with fears about its potential effects

Outcome measurement criteria

- ☐ Verbalization of accurate knowledge about the condition
- ☐ Acknowledgment of the need for treatment
- ☐ Acknowledgment and discussion of concerns
- ☐ Demonstration of appropriate range of feelings

Key interventions

- Maintain a calm, professional demeanor at the bedside and with family members.
- Assess the patient's and family's emotional reaction to the condition.
- Help the patient and family understand information about the condition and the need for treatment.
- Keep the patient and family informed about maternal and fetal status.
- Within the limitations imposed by resuscitative efforts, explain procedures to the patient and family.
- Help the patient and family identify and use available resources (such as other family members, other health care professionals, and clergy) to promote discussion of feelings.

NURSING DIAGNOSIS

High risk for fluid volume deficit related to excessive blood loss secondary to altered clotting mechanism

DESIRED PATIENT OUTCOME

The patient will maintain adequate fluid volume and electrolyte balance

Outcome measurement criteria

☐ No signs of hemorrhage

☐ Blood pressure within normal range for the patient

☐ Urine output greater than or equal to 30 ml/hour

☐ Electrolyte values within normal ranges

☐ Coagulation study results within normal ranges

☐ Hemodynamic monitoring values within normal ranges

Key interventions

- Monitor and document the patient's vital signs.

- Assess for signs of a clotting disorder, such as epistaxis and bleeding from injection sites. Report such findings immediately.

- Assist with evaluating electrolyte and coagulation studies.

- Assist with inserting internal monitoring devices, as required.

- Administer I.V. fluids, medications, and blood components as prescribed.

- Monitor and document fluid intake and output and the patient's hemodynamic status.

NURSING DIAGNOSIS

High risk for infection related to the use of invasive monitoring devices

DESIRED PATIENT OUTCOME

The patient will not develop an infection due to invasive monitoring

Outcome measurement criteria

☐ Oral temperature at or below 100.4° F (38° C)

☐ White blood cell (WBC) count within normal range

☐ Absence of localized erythema, edema, and warmth at insertion sites

☐ No signs or symptoms of urinary tract infection (UTI)

Key interventions

- Assess and document vital signs. Examine the patient for signs of systemic or local infection.

- Evaluate laboratory study results as indicated, particularly noting the WBC count.

- Reassess the insertion sites periodically to detect signs of infection, such as localized erythema, edema, and warmth. Also assess for signs and symptoms of UTI, such as dysuria, hematuria, and urinary frequency and urgency.

- Maintain asepsis and hand-washing practices. Teach these practices to the patient and family members as indicated.

Cesarean delivery

Extraction of the infant, amniotic fluid, and placenta through surgical incisions in the maternal abdomen and uterus.

NURSING DIAGNOSIS

Fear related to perceived threat to self and lack of knowledge about cesarean delivery

DESIRED PATIENT OUTCOME

The patient and family will express decreased fear and increased satisfaction with the plan for cesarean delivery

Outcome measurement criteria

☐ Acknowledgment of the need for cesarean delivery

☐ Expression of accurate knowledge about the procedures involved in cesarean delivery

☐ Expression of accurate knowledge of maternal and fetal risks and benefits

☐ Verbalization of accurate knowledge about the anticipated postoperative course

☐ Verbalization of feelings about cesarean delivery

Key interventions

• Assess the patient's and family's level of knowledge about cesarean delivery. Encourage them to express their feelings and concerns.

• Help the patient and family obtain accurate information about the procedure. Encourage them to ask questions; provide accurate information and correct any misconceptions.

- Teach the patient and family about preoperative preparation. Explain the various aspects of surgical preparation.

- Discuss postoperative care, including surgical wound care, activity limitations, wound splinting, pain relief, vital sign monitoring, and measures to promote oxygenation.

- Verify the patient's and family's understanding of the information provided.

NURSING DIAGNOSIS

Situational low self-esteem related to failure to accomplish vaginal delivery

DESIRED PATIENT OUTCOME

The patient will report restored self-esteem

Outcome measurement criteria

☐ Acknowledgment of the unavoidability of cesarean delivery

☐ Identification of positive aspects of labor and delivery

☐ Expression of satisfaction with cesarean delivery

☐ Verbalization of positive expectations for future deliveries

Key interventions

- Assess the patient's feelings about the cesarean delivery. Encourage her to express these feelings.

- Discuss the patient's expectations for labor and delivery and the ways in which the actual labor and delivery were similar to and different from those expectations.

- Help the patient accept negative and positive feelings about labor and delivery.

- Reinforce the rationale for proceeding with cesarean delivery. Encourage the patient to accept the situation and avoid blaming herself or others.

- Encourage the patient to explore plans for future deliveries, if desired, and help her to focus on positive expectations.

- For related information, see "Postpartal common course" in the Postpartal Period section.

Dystocia

Excessively painful, prolonged, or difficult labor or delivery due to such conditions as hypotonic uterine activity, hypertonic uterine activity, maternal soft tissue obstruction of the birth passage, fetal malpresentation, or fetal shoulder impaction.

NURSING DIAGNOSIS

Pain related to intense uterine contractions or prolonged labor

DESIRED PATIENT OUTCOME

The patient will report relief or toleration of pain associated with uterine contractions

Outcome measurement criteria

☐ Communication of the need for assistance with managing pain

☐ Appearance of relaxation between contractions

☐ Appropriate use of pharmacologic and nonpharmacologic pain-relief methods

☐ Report of decreased or tolerable pain

Key interventions

- Assess the patient's level and tolerance of pain.

- Teach the patient about the nature of uterine contraction pain. Use an electronic monitor to demonstrate the increment, acme, and decrement phases of a uterine contraction.

- Reassure the patient about the temporary nature of contraction pain.

- Take measures to increase physical comfort, such as providing support with pillows, applying cool damp cloths to the forehead, performing back rubs, and repositioning the patient in bed at intervals.

- As appropriate, encourage the patient to ambulate to decrease physical discomfort from prolonged bed rest and to increase the effects of gravity on dilation and effacement.

- Teach the patient appropriate communication methods and reinforce her use of these methods. Help the patient accurately identify and communicate her specific needs for assistance with pain relief, such as a pillow for her back, repositioning in bed, relocation of an external monitor, or analgesics.

- Help the patient use relaxation techniques to relieve pain. Also encourage her to physically relax as much as possible between and during contractions. Reinforce her efforts toward relaxation.

- Offer pharmacologic pain-relief methods as prescribed. Teach the patient about available choices for pain relief during labor.

- Administer analgesics as prescribed. Assist with preparation for anesthesia administration as ordered.

NURSING DIAGNOSIS

Ineffective individual coping related to ineffective breathing patterns, fatigue, fear, or lack of adequate support during labor and delivery

DESIRED PATIENT OUTCOME

The patient will demonstrate effective coping behaviors throughout labor and delivery

Outcome measurement criteria

☐ Absence of hyperventilation

☐ Use of various effective breathing patterns

☐ Verbalization of physical ability to continue labor

☐ Expression of specific concerns related to the outcome of labor

☐ Verbalization of accurate understanding of maternal and fetal well-being

☐ Presence of effective support person throughout labor

Key interventions

• Assess the patient's coping behaviors during labor. Identify ineffective or inappropriate coping behaviors and reinforce effective ones.

• Discourage the use of inappropriate coping behaviors, such as thrashing in bed, abusive language, and physical violence. Teach the patient alternative behaviors.

• Encourage the patient to use positive coping techniques, such as visualization, distraction, and focusing.

• Help the patient recognize ineffective breathing patterns, such as hyperventilation. Demonstrate various breathing patterns that can be used during contractions to promote adequate gas exchange. Encourage the patient to control her breathing.

• Decrease the potential for fatigue by providing a restful environment. Organize care to decrease the frequency of interruptions to the resting patient. Encourage her to rest as much as possible during labor.

• Administer I.V. fluids as prescribed and offer high carbohydrate juices and candies as ordered to increase blood glucose levels for rapidly available energy.

• Encourage the patient and family to verbalize fears and concerns about dystocia and its potential effects on maternal and fetal well-being.

- Help the patient and family understand actual and potential risks to the mother and fetus resulting from dystocia.

- Frequently inform the patient and family members of the patient's progress in labor. Offer frequent encouragement and reassurance about progress. Help the patient and family recognize even small changes in cervical effacement and dilation and station of the presenting part as significant changes.

- Acknowledge the importance of positive support people. Reinforce the need for continued presence of a support person with patient. Relieve the support person as needed and remain with the patient as indicated.

NURSING DIAGNOSIS

Situational low self-esteem related to inability to complete labor and delivery as planned

DESIRED PATIENT OUTCOME

The patient will maintain a positive self-concept throughout labor and delivery

Outcome measurement criteria

☐ Absence of expressions of shame or guilt

☐ Verbalization of positive self-appraisal

☐ Verbalization of understanding of unavoidability of dystocia

Key interventions

- Encourage the patient to discuss her feelings about differences between her imagined course of labor and the actual course of labor.

- Be alert for indications of self-esteem disturbances, such as statements of negative self-appraisal or feelings of failure.

- Teach the patient that most women discover that the fantasized course of labor and delivery is not like the actual labor and delivery.

- Encourage the patient to acknowledge the unavoidability of dystocia.

- Acknowledge positive factors related to the patient's labor and delivery, such as her preparedness for labor and use of effective coping techniques and the infant's health at birth. Encourage the patient to recognize these as significant.

NURSING DIAGNOSIS

High risk for fluid volume deficit related to restricted oral intake, vomiting, and increased insensible fluid loss during prolonged labor

DESIRED PATIENT OUTCOME

The patient will maintain adequate fluid volume and electrolyte balance throughout labor and delivery

Outcome measurement criteria

☐ Blood pressure within normal range for patient

☐ Skin warm to touch and without mottling or cyanosis

☐ Moist mucous membranes

☐ Urine output greater than or equal to 30 ml/hour

☐ Absence of ketones in urine

☐ Urine specific gravity of 1.003 to 1.030

☐ Electrolyte levels within normal ranges

Key interventions

- Monitor and document the patient's vital signs.

- Assess the moistness of the mucous membranes. Provide oral care to moisten dry oral mucous membranes.

- Administer I.V. and oral fluids as prescribed.

- Monitor and document fluid intake and output.

- Encourage the patient to void at least every 2 hours.

- Report ketonuria or urine specific gravity that does not fall within the normal range. Report other abnormal laboratory results to the health care professional.

- Encourage controlled breathing to decrease insensible fluid loss.

- Alter the room temperature to improve the patient's comfort and decrease fluid loss through diaphoresis.

NURSING DIAGNOSIS

High risk for infection related to invasive monitoring and frequent assessment

DESIRED PATIENT OUTCOME

The patient will remain free from infection caused by invasive monitoring and frequent assessment

Outcome measurement criteria

- ☐ Oral temperature at or below 100.4° F (38° C)

- ☐ Absence of malodorous amniotic fluid

- ☐ Absence of erythema, edema, and warmth at insertion sites of monitoring devices

- ☐ No signs or symptoms of urinary tract infection

- ☐ Absence of foul-smelling lochia

- ☐ Absence of purulent drainage from episiotomy site or surgical wound

☐ Absence of extreme postpartal uterine tenderness

☐ White blood cell (WBC) count within normal postpartal range

Key interventions

- Use strict sterile technique for vaginal examinations and insertion of invasive monitoring devices.

- Minimize the number of vaginal examinations.

- Monitor and document vital signs. Assess the patient's temperature at least once every 4 hours.

- If a fever is suspected, monitor the patient's temperature every 1 to 2 hours. Report significant changes to the health care professional.

- Change the bed linens as indicated to decrease the patient's risk of exposure to pathogens.

- Maintain asepsis and strict hand-washing practices. Teach these practices to the patient and family members as indicated.

- Assess amniotic fluid for odor. Notify the health care professional if a foul odor develops.

- Assess for dysuria. Encourage voiding at least every 2 hours for the first 12 hours after removal of an indwelling urinary (Foley) catheter.

- Assess the episiotomy or surgical wound site for signs of infection, such as purulent drainage, excessive erythema, edema, redness, and poor approximation.

- Assess for extreme postpartal uterine tenderness and malodorous lochia.

- Assist with interpreting the WBC as ordered and report abnormal findings.

NURSING DIAGNOSIS

High risk for injury (maternal) related to soft tissue damage secondary to difficult labor and delivery

DESIRED PATIENT OUTCOME

The patient will not sustain injury from soft tissue damage

Outcome measurement criteria

☐ Absence of cervical lacerations

☐ Absence of perianal or periurethral lacerations

☐ Absence of third- or fourth-degree perineal lacerations

Key interventions

- Encourage the patient to avoid pushing prematurely if cervical edema occurs in the transition phase of labor. Instead, help her avoid pushing by using breathing techniques, such as panting.

- Encourage the use of controlled pushing techniques to avoid traumatic damage to perianal, periurethral, and perineal tissue.

- Assist with techniques to rotate the fetus from an occiput posterior presentation to an occiput anterior presentation to decrease the risk of soft tissue damage. Encourage the use of the knee-chest or hands-and-knees position for labor and pushing as indicated.

- Encourage the patient to concentrate on relaxing her pelvic floor musculature. Palpate the pelvic floor musculature to help her identify effective relaxation. Tell the patient when the musculature becomes too taut.

- Use pelvic floor stretching techniques as indicated.

NURSING DIAGNOSIS

High risk for injury (fetal) related to prolonged compression against maternal pelvic structures, decreased uteroplacental circulation, or shoulder dystocia

DESIRED PATIENT OUTCOME

The fetus will not sustain injury during labor or delivery

Outcome measurement criteria

☐ No indications of fetal hypoxia during labor

☐ Absence of soft tissue injury

☐ Absence of skeletal fractures

☐ Absence of neuromuscular damage

☐ Absence of central nervous system (CNS) damage

☐ Delivery of a viable, noninjured infant

Key interventions

• Identify a fetus at risk as early as possible in labor by noting predisposing factors (macrosomia, a prolonged second stage of labor, multiparity, prolonged pregnancy, and previous birth of an infant weighing more than 4,000 g [8.8 lb]) and estimating fetal size, lie, and presentation. Notify the health care professional if assessment reveals fetal malpresentation.

• Monitor the fetal heart rate throughout labor and delivery. Be alert for nonreassuring patterns. Notify the health care professional if nonreassuring patterns occur.

• Note the presence or absence of molding on vaginal examination. On subsequent assessments, note and document any change in the character of the molding.

• For a fetus with shoulder dystocia, use McRoberts maneuver to alter the angle of the maternal pelvis and decrease the risk of brachial plexus or clavicular damage to the infant. Help the patient fully flex her hips and legs and pull her knees toward her shoulders while lifting her head toward her abdomen.

- Assess for signs of injury upon delivery of the infant. Notify the health care professional of any soft tissue injury, skeletal fractures, or neuromuscular or CNS damage.

Eclampsia

A severe pregnancy complication characterized by tonic and clonic seizures, hypertension, oliguria, and proteinuria.

NURSING DIAGNOSIS

High risk for injury (maternal and fetal) related to the effects of seizures

DESIRED PATIENT OUTCOME

The patient and fetus will remain free from injury caused by seizures

Outcome measurement criteria

☐ Absence of maternal soft tissue damage

☐ Respiratory rate of 12 to 20 breaths/minute

☐ Blood pressure within normal range

☐ Urine output greater than or equal to 30 ml/hour

☐ Absence of nonreassuring fetal heart rate (FHR) pattern

☐ Delivery of a viable infant

Key interventions

• Maintain the environment to decrease central nervous system stimulation; for example, turn off bright lights, speak quietly to the patient and support person, turn off televisions and radios, and control the amount of noise outside the patient's room.

• Take seizure precautions during patient care. Pad the side rails of the bed. Keep oxygen and an airway at the patient's bedside.

- Monitor and document the duration and nature of seizures.
- Administer medications and I.V. fluids as prescribed.
- Monitor and document vital signs.
- Assess fluid intake and output.
- Continually assess fetal status, particularly the FHR.
- Assist with supportive therapy while preparing for delivery.

NURSING DIAGNOSIS
Altered fetal tissue perfusion related to a rapid decrease in available oxygen secondary to maternal seizures

DESIRED PATIENT OUTCOME
The patient will maintain sufficient placental circulation of oxygenated blood to support fetal life

Outcome measurement criteria
☐ FHR of 120 to 160 beats/minute
☐ Average long-term variability of FHR
☐ No nonreassuring FHR patterns
☐ FHR accelerations with fetal movement
☐ Delivery of a viable infant

Key interventions
- Administer oxygen by tight face mask after a seizure as prescribed to promote fetal oxygenation.
- Position the patient to promote optimum placental circulation.
- Continually monitor and document the FHR. Be alert for changes in variability and nonreassuring patterns.

- Notify the health care professional of nonreassuring FHR patterns.

NURSING DIAGNOSIS

High risk for aspiration related to seizures

DESIRED PATIENT OUTCOME

The patient will not experience aspiration caused by seizures

Outcome measurement criteria

☐ Airway free of obstruction

☐ Respiratory rate of 12 to 20 breaths/minute

☐ Lungs clear on auscultation

☐ Absence of signs and symptoms of hypoxia

Key interventions

- Position the patient laterally (preferably on the left side) during and after seizures.
- Suction the patient's airway after a seizure to remove obstructions.
- Assess for return of spontaneous respiration after a seizure stops.
- Assess the patient's lung sounds. Maintain a clear airway by repeated suctioning as needed.
- Administer oxygen as prescribed.
- Perform resuscitative efforts as indicated.

NURSING DIAGNOSIS

High risk for fluid volume deficit related to excessive blood loss secondary to complications of eclampsia

DESIRED PATIENT OUTCOME

The patient will maintain adequate fluid volume and electrolyte balance

Outcome measurement criteria

☐ Blood pressure within normal range for patient

☐ No narrowing of pulse pressure

☐ Pulse rate of 60 to 90 beats/minute

☐ Palpable peripheral pulses

☐ Skin warm to touch and without mottling or cyanosis

☐ No confusion or loss of consciousness

☐ Urine output greater than or equal to 30 ml/hour

☐ Electrolyte and blood component values within normal ranges

☐ Coagulation study results within normal ranges

☐ Hemodynamic monitoring values within normal ranges

Key interventions

• Monitor and document vital signs.

• Assess for signs of a developing clotting disorder, such as epistaxis and bleeding from injection sites. Document and report findings immediately.

• Assess and document level of consciousness.

• Administer I.V. fluids, medications, and blood components as prescribed.

• Assist with evaluation of laboratory tests.

• Assist with insertion of internal monitoring devices as required.

• Monitor and document fluid intake and output and the patient's hemodynamic status.

• Initiate and assist with resuscitative efforts as indicated.

NURSING DIAGNOSIS

High risk for infection related to use of invasive monitoring and vaginal examinations

DESIRED PATIENT OUTCOME

The patient will not develop an infection from invasive monitoring and vaginal examinations

Outcome measurement criteria

☐ Oral temperature at or below 100.4° F (38° C)

☐ White blood cell (WBC) count within normal range

☐ Absence of localized erythema, edema, and warmth at insertion sites of monitoring devices

☐ No signs or symptoms of urinary tract infection

Key interventions

• Monitor and document vital signs. Assess for signs and symptoms of systemic and local infection.

• Evaluate laboratory test results for an increasing WBC count and decreasing erythrocyte sedimentation rate.

• Maintain asepsis and hand-washing practices. Teach appropriate practices to the patient and family members as indicated.

NURSING DIAGNOSIS

Fear related to lack of knowledge about eclampsia's treatment and its potential effects on maternal and fetal well-being

DESIRED PATIENT OUTCOME

The patient and family will express increased knowledge about treatments for eclampsia and cope effectively with fears about its potential effects

Outcome measurement criteria

☐ Verbalization of accurate knowledge of eclampsia

☐ Acknowledgment of the need for treatment

☐ Acknowledgment and discussion of concerns

☐ Demonstration of appropriate affect

Key interventions

- Maintain a calm, professional demeanor at the bedside and with family members.

- Assess the patient's and family's emotional reaction to the condition.

- Help the patient and family obtain accurate information about eclampsia and the need for treatment.

- Keep the patient and family informed of maternal and fetal status.

- Explain procedures to the patient and family as much as possible, using short, clear statements.

- Help the patient and family identify and use available resources (such as other family members, other health care professionals, clergy, and support groups) to promote discussion of feelings.

Electronic fetal monitoring

The use of electronic instruments to assess fetal heart rate (FHR) patterns and uterine contractions.

NURSING DIAGNOSIS
Anxiety related to lack of knowledge about electronic fetal monitoring

DESIRED PATIENT OUTCOME
The patient and family will appear relaxed and express increased knowledge about electronic fetal monitoring

Outcome measurement criteria
☐ Absence of signs of anxiety

☐ Expression of satisfaction with plan for using an electronic fetal monitor

☐ Expression of accurate understanding of how and why electronic fetal monitoring is done

☐ Expression of accurate understanding of gross interpretation of fetal monitor patterns

Key interventions
• Assess the patient's and family's knowledge of how and why to use an electronic fetal monitor. Correct misconceptions as needed.

• Teach the patient and family about the anticipated procedure. Explain what is expected of the patient and the health care team members throughout monitoring.

- Teach the patient and family about general interpretation of fetal monitor patterns; for example, explain that the monitor is used to determine how the fetus is affected by labor. The fetus's ability to change its heart rate in response to activity is an indication of well-being.

- Teach the patient and family that the monitor also will be used to track uterine activity. Explain that the monitor evaluates the frequency and duration of contractions.

- Encourage the patient and family to ask questions.

NURSING DIAGNOSIS

Pain related to the perceived need to remain immobile and the presence of monitor attachments

DESIRED PATIENT OUTCOME

The patient will experience little or no pain from electronic fetal monitoring

Outcome measurement criteria

☐ Verbalization of accurate understanding of acceptable activity levels during monitoring

☐ Acknowledgment of the need for monitor attachments

☐ Appropriate communication of needs

☐ Report of little or no pain

Key interventions

- Assess the patient's level of knowledge about monitor placement and acceptable activities during monitoring.

- Teach the patient about the appropriate placement of a tocotransducer, external FHR monitor, internal scalp electrode, and intrauterine pressure catheter, as indicated.

- Encourage the patient to report pain or discomfort that results from monitor placement. Reassure her that monitoring should not cause pain.

- Teach the patient that movement in bed is acceptable during monitoring. Caution the patient against feeling the need to remain completely still.

- Encourage the patient to communicate her need for help with repositioning herself in bed.

NURSING DIAGNOSIS
High risk for injury (fetal) related to hypoxia secondary to persistent nonreassuring FHR patterns or the absence of uterine resting tone

DESIRED PATIENT OUTCOME
The fetus will not sustain injury from hypoxia during labor

Outcome measurement criteria
- ☐ Palpation of soft uterine resting tone between contractions
- ☐ Uterine resting tone of less than 15 mm Hg when using an intrauterine pressure catheter
- ☐ FHR baseline of 120 to 160 beats/minute
- ☐ Average short-term variability (STV) and long-term variability (LTV) in FHR
- ☐ FHR accelerations with fetal movement
- ☐ FHR acceleration of 15 beats/minute for 15 seconds after scalp stimulation
- ☐ Absence of persistent variable or late decelerations
- ☐ Absence of persistent fetal bradycardia or tachycardia
- ☐ Fetal scalp blood pH greater than 7.20

☐ Delivery of a viable infant

Key interventions

- Ensure that the monitoring equipment is working properly. Assess the suitability of plugs and wires, accuracy of paper insertion in the monitor, availability of ultrasound transmission gel, and availability of external and internal monitoring devices.

- Frequently check for accurate placement of monitors on and in the patient. Document changes in placement of monitoring devices.

- Frequently assess and document maternal vital signs, maternal activity, and periodic changes in FHR. Also document interventions, especially medication administration.

- Assess and document uterine resting tone. If resting tone is absent, discontinue oxytocin (Pitocin) as indicated, reposition the patient, and notify the health care professional.

- Assess the patient's temperature for elevation if fetal tachycardia persists.

- Reposition the patient for improved uteroplacental circulation if fetal bradycardia persists. Verify the accuracy of the FHR by counting the maternal heart rate. Apply an internal scalp electrode as indicated to more accurately assess FHR.

- Assess and document STV and LTV. Anticipate decreased STV and LTV after administration of analgesics and anesthetics.

- If STV is minimal to absent, assess for reassuring FHR patterns by performing scalp stimulation as needed.

- If variable decelerations persist, administer warmed fluid by amnioinfusion as prescribed to cushion the umbilical cord against compression from contractions.

- Notify the health care professional if assessment reveals suspicious, threatening, ominous, or chronic nonreassuring FHR patterns.

- If a nonreassuring FHR pattern occurs, be prepared to perform intrauterine resuscitation: Change the maternal position to improve maternal or uteroplacental circulation; discontinue the oxytocin infusion to decrease contraction frequency, intensity, and duration; increase the I.V. fluid infusion rate to increase maternal circulating volume; and administer oxygen by tight face mask at 10 liters/minute to increase placental oxygen flow.

- Assist with fetal scalp blood sampling as ordered.

- Assist with preparation for emergency cesarean delivery as indicated.

- Keep the patient and family informed. Use short, clear sentences when explaining the reason for preventive or emergency procedures.

HELLP syndrome

A life-threatening variant of preeclampsia involving physiologic changes that produce hemolysis, elevated liver enzymes, and a low platelet count.

NURSING DIAGNOSIS

High risk for injury (maternal and fetal) related to abnormal cardiovascular function and multisystem organ dysfunction secondary to HELLP syndrome

DESIRED PATIENT OUTCOME

The patient and fetus will remain free of injury during the intrapartal and postpartal periods

Outcome measurement criteria

- ☐ Stable maternal blood pressure
- ☐ Urine output greater than or equal to 30 ml/hour
- ☐ Stable or improved laboratory test results, including complete blood count, platelet count, and electrolyte, liver enzyme, and coagulation component levels
- ☐ Serum magnesium level within therapeutic range
- ☐ Absence of eclamptic seizures
- ☐ Absence of hemorrhage
- ☐ Absence of pulmonary edema
- ☐ Hemodynamic monitoring values within normal ranges
- ☐ Reactive nonstress test results
- ☐ Presence of long-term fetal heart rate variability
- ☐ Delivery of a viable infant

Key interventions

- Monitor and document vital signs, urine output, lung sounds, and hemodynamic status.

- Assess the patient for increasing edema and blood pressure, severe headache, decreasing urine output, epigastric pain, severe nausea and vomiting, decreased or absent reflexes, dyspnea, adventitious lung sounds, and abnormal bleeding tendencies. Document and report findings.

- Maintain a controlled environment to decrease the patient's central nervous system stimulation. For example, provide a quiet, dark atmosphere and organize nursing care to decrease the number of interruptions to the patient.

- Assist with evaluation of hemodynamic status and laboratory values.

- Conduct fetal evaluation as ordered. Note evidence of fetal well-being or distress on the fetal monitor in non-stress testing or during labor.

- Administer I.V. fluids, magnesium sulfate, blood products, corticosteroids, and other medications as prescribed.

- Plan to assess closely for postpartal uterine involution.

NURSING DIAGNOSIS

Fear related to lack of knowledge about treatment for HELLP syndrome and the disorder's potential effects on maternal and fetal well-being

DESIRED PATIENT OUTCOME

The patient and family will express increased knowledge about treatments for HELLP and will cope effectively with fears about its potential effects

Outcome measurement criteria

☐ Verbalization of accurate knowledge of the disorder

☐ Acknowledgment of the need for treatment

☐ Acknowledgment and discussion of concerns

☐ Demonstration of appropriate affect

Key interventions

- Maintain a calm, professional demeanor at the bedside and with family members.

- Assess the patient's and family's emotional reaction to the disorder.

- Help the patient and family obtain accurate information about HELLP syndrome and the need for treatment.

- Keep the patient and family informed about maternal and fetal status throughout labor and delivery.

- Explain all procedures to the patient and family.

NURSING DIAGNOSIS

High risk for dysfunctional grieving related to maternal and fetal morbidity and possible mortality secondary to HELLP syndrome

DESIRED PATIENT OUTCOME

The patient and family will progress through the stages of grief and will express hope for the future

Outcome measurement criteria

☐ Acknowledgment of the effect of this loss on self and family

☐ Absence of self-blame

☐ Engagement in appropriate self-care activities

☐ Use of external resources as needed

Key interventions

- Establish a therapeutic relationship with the patient and family and validate the reality of the loss. When the patient is ready, discuss the stages of grief.

- Encourage the patient and family to discuss their feelings about the effect of the loss.

- Encourage the family to accept and recognize differences in individual and cultural responses to grief.

- Stress the importance of avoiding self-blame. Encourage the patient and family to recognize that the physiologic alterations that occur with this syndrome are beyond their control.

- Teach appropriate self-care measures for the intrapartal period. Allow time for rest to promote emotional and physical recovery.

- Provide information about support groups, counselors, clergy, or telephone hotlines for the patient and family. Encourage use of these or other resources if they have difficulty resolving grief.

NURSING DIAGNOSIS

Altered family processes related to the effects of a critical maternal and fetal illness

DESIRED PATIENT OUTCOME

The patient and family will adapt positively to changes imposed by maternal and fetal illness

Outcome measurement criteria

- ☐ Open expression of feelings about the effects of HELLP syndrome on the family

- ☐ Expression of understanding of the disorder and its treatment and prognosis

☐ Participation in plans for solving family problems arising from the disorder, such as difficulties managing finances, caring for children, and performing household duties.

☐ Use of appropriate resources for help in resolving family problems

Key interventions

• Encourage the family to ask questions and verbalize concerns. Help the family obtain accurate information about the disorder's severity and treatment and the prognosis for the mother and fetus.

• Encourage open expression of feelings but reinforce the need to limit stress on the patient. Encourage family members to seek alternative outlets for discussing fears and concerns as needed.

• Help mobilize known support systems, such as extended family, friends, church groups, support groups, and clergy.

• Provide written and verbal information about resources that may be unknown to the family. Provide a referral for social services as indicated.

• Help the family examine the effect of the disorder on their usual family processes, including financial implications and changes in role expectations.

NURSING DIAGNOSIS

High risk for infection related to the use of an invasive monitoring device

DESIRED PATIENT OUTCOME

The patient will not develop infection caused by an invasive monitoring device

Outcome measurement criteria

☐ Oral temperature at or below 100.4° F (38° C)

☐ White blood cell count within normal range

☐ Absence of localized erythema, edema, and warmth at insertion sites of monitoring devices

☐ No signs or symptoms of urinary tract infection

Key interventions

• Monitor and document vital signs. Assess for signs and symptoms of systemic and local infection.

• Report findings of laboratory studies as ordered.

• Maintain asepsis and strict hand-washing practices. Teach these practices to the patient and family members as indicated.

Induction of labor

Deliberate stimulation or augmentation of labor through oxytocin or prostaglandin administration or nipple stimulation.

NURSING DIAGNOSIS
Anxiety related to lack of knowledge about labor induction

DESIRED PATIENT OUTCOME
The patient and family will appear relaxed and express increased knowledge about labor induction

Outcome measurement criteria
☐ Absence of signs of anxiety
☐ Expression of satisfaction with the plan for labor induction
☐ Acknowledgment of the need for labor induction
☐ Expression of an accurate understanding of anticipated procedures
☐ Verbalization of anticipated outcomes of procedures

Key interventions
• Assess the patient's and family's knowledge of the planned method of labor induction.
• Help the patient and family obtain accurate information about labor induction. Correct misconceptions as needed.
• Teach the patient and family about the labor induction procedure. Explain anticipated activities of the patient, fetus, and health care team members during induction.

- Encourage the patient and family to ask questions.
- Verify their understanding of the information presented. Provide written documentation as needed.
- Verify documentation of informed consent before labor induction begins.

NURSING DIAGNOSIS

High risk for situational low self-esteem related to feelings of failure secondary to the need for labor induction

DESIRED PATIENT OUTCOME

The patient will express restored self-esteem

Outcome measurement criteria

☐ Acknowledgment of the unavoidability of the need for labor induction

☐ Identification of positive aspects of labor induction

☐ Expression of understanding that labor induction commonly is required

☐ Verbalization of positive expectations for self in the maternal role

Key interventions

- Assess the patient's feelings about labor induction and encourage her to express these feelings.
- Help the patient accept her negative and positive feelings about labor and delivery.
- Encourage the patient to talk about her expectations of labor and delivery. Help her recognize that induction can assist in meeting her expectations.
- Explain the scientific rationale for proceeding with labor induction. Reinforce the unavoidability of induction.

- Encourage the patient to discuss her expectations about her maternal role. Help her focus on positive self-expectations.

NURSING DIAGNOSIS

High risk for altered placental tissue perfusion related to uterine hyperstimulation caused by labor induction

DESIRED PATIENT OUTCOME

The patient will maintain adequate placental perfusion

Outcome measurement criteria

☐ Fetal heart rate (FHR) of 120 to 160 beats/minute

☐ Average short-term variability and long-term variability in FHR

☐ No nonreassuring FHR patterns

☐ FHR accelerations with fetal movement

☐ Contractions not more frequent than every 2½ to 3 minutes

☐ Contractions not longer than 90 seconds each

☐ Soft uterine resting tone between contractions

☐ Delivery of a viable infant

Key interventions

- Before labor induction, evaluate the patient and fetus for contraindications, such as previous classical uterine incision, fetal malpresentation, and prematurity.
- Monitor and document the FHR, particularly noting variability and nonreassuring patterns.
- Document and report nonreassuring patterns or absence of variability.

- Reposition the patient as needed to promote optimum uteroplacental circulation. Use the left lateral (most preferred), right lateral, or semi-Fowler's position; avoid the supine position because it can lead to vena cava syndrome.

- Monitor and document uterine activity. Be alert for marked increases in contraction frequency, intensity, and duration.

- Discontinue I.V. oxytocin if nonreassuring FHR patterns or signs of uterine hyperstimulation occur.

- Administer oxygen at 8 to 10 liters/minute by tight face mask as prescribed to promote increased fetal oxygenation.

- Administer a warmed I.V. fluid bolus as prescribed to reduce adverse reactions to labor induction.

Infections

Infections caused by organisms that may cross the placental barrier and cause serious fetal damage.

NURSING DIAGNOSIS
High risk for infection (fetal) related to human immuno-deficiency virus (HIV) exposure from the mother

DESIRED PATIENT OUTCOME
The patient will minimize the risk of HIV transmission to her fetus during delivery

Outcome measurement criteria
☐ Verbalization of ways to help prevent HIV transmission to the fetus

☐ Use of techniques to prevent HIV transmission by the patient, family, and health care team members

Key interventions
- Advocate avoiding artificial rupture of membranes during labor. Document the time of membrane rupture and the appearance, quantity, and odor of amniotic fluid. Communicate this information to the health care professional.

- Advocate the use of external fetal monitoring rather than invasive monitoring, such as via fetal scalp elec-trodes and blood sampling, during labor to decrease the risk of direct transmission to the fetus via contact with body fluids.

- Explain the use of protective barriers in the hospital to decrease the risk of transmission to the infant. Use universal precautions when handling the infant.

- Instruct the patient to avoid breast-feeding, because HIV has been isolated in breast milk and may increase the infant's risk of exposure.

- Assist with suctioning the infant's nares and oropharynx on emergence from the birth canal.

- Bathe the infant with soap and water before administering injected medications.

NURSING DIAGNOSIS

High risk for infection (fetal) related to exposure to organisms that cause TORCH infections from the pregnant patient

DESIRED PATIENT OUTCOME

The patient will take actions to prevent infection of her fetus

Outcome measurement criteria

☐ Use of techniques to avoid infection by the pregnant patient and her family and health care team members

☐ Absence of signs of infection in the infant

Key interventions

- Advocate avoiding artificial rupture of membranes during labor. Document the time of membrane rupture and the appearance, quantity, and odor of amniotic fluid. Communicate this information to the health care professional.

- Advocate the use of external fetal monitoring rather than invasive monitoring, such as via fetal scalp electrodes and blood sampling, during labor to decrease the risk of disease transmission to the fetus.

- Inform the patient that protective barriers will be used in the hospital to decrease the risk of infecting the infant. Use universal precautions when handling the infant.

- Assist with preparation for surgical delivery as needed to decrease the risk of disease transmission to the fetus. Reassure and comfort the patient throughout this preparation.

- Assist with suctioning the infant's nares and oropharynx on emergence from the birth canal.

- Bathe the infant with soap and water before administering injected medications. Let alcohol dry on the infant's skin for 1 full minute before injection to decrease the risk of contamination via needle puncture.

Labor and vaginal delivery, common course

Processes by which the products of conception are expelled from the uterus. They occur in four stages:

- *The first stage, which has latent, active, and transition phases, includes the beginning of cervical dilation and fetal descent.*
- *The second stage, which also has latent, active, and transition phases, extends from complete cervical dilation to delivery of the infant.*
- *The third stage extends from delivery of the infant to delivery of the placenta.*
- *The fourth stage includes the initial physiologic recovery and emotional bonding that occur in the first several hours after delivery of the infant.*

NURSING DIAGNOSIS
Fear related to unfamiliarity with labor

DESIRED PATIENT OUTCOME
The patient will express decreased fear of labor and increased satisfaction with the plan of care

Outcome measurement criteria
- ☐ Expression of familiarity with physical surroundings
- ☐ Expression of an accurate understanding of the anticipated course of labor
- ☐ Verbalization of accurate knowledge of the anticipated nursing actions during labor
- ☐ Report of satisfaction with the plan of care

☐ Communication of needs for assistance throughout labor

Key interventions

- Orient the patient to the physical surroundings in the labor area. Teach her how to use the call button, bed, television, and other equipment in the room as needed.

- Assess the patient's expectations for labor. Assess her plans for use of anesthesia or analgesia, various breathing techniques, pain-relief methods, positions for labor and delivery, and the planned role for the support person. Incorporate the patient's wishes into the plan of care as much as possible.

- Briefly explain the use of the electronic fetal monitor, if used.

- Briefly explain what the patient can expect during the normal course of labor, including anticipated time intervals between the onset of labor and delivery of the infant.

- Reassure the patient that her comfort is important during labor. Teach her about limitations on moving about freely during labor.

- Encourage mobility as much as possible. Have the patient ambulate or shower or sit up in bed during the latent phase of labor and during the active and transition phases, if possible.

- Briefly explain the rationale for administration of I.V. fluid, if used.

- Teach about typical nursing actions during the normal course of labor, including monitoring contractions and fetal heart rate (FHR), starting and maintaining an I.V. line, performing vaginal examinations, monitoring vital signs, and supporting the patient and family members.

- Encourage the patient to communicate her needs to health care team members as labor progresses.

- Determine if plans for labor management meet the patient's expectations. Modify plans, if possible, to meet specific patient needs that arise during labor.

NURSING DIAGNOSIS

Pain related to increasing intensity and duration of uterine contractions

DESIRED PATIENT OUTCOME

The patient will report increased comfort or a tolerable level of pain caused by uterine contractions

Outcome measurement criteria

☐ Appropriate communication of need for assistance with pain relief

☐ Appearance of relaxation between contractions

☐ Use of pharmacologic and nonpharmacologic pain-relief methods

☐ Report of decreased or tolerable pain

Key interventions

- Assess the patient's level of pain. Teach her about the nature of pain from contractions. Use the electronic monitor to demonstrate increment, acme, and decrement phases of uterine contractions.

- Reassure the patient that pain from contractions is temporary.

- Take measures to increase the patient's physical comfort. For example, support her with pillows, apply cool damp cloths to her forehead, perform backrubs, and reposition her in bed regularly.

- Help the patient identify and communicate specific needs for assistance with pain relief, such as a pillow to her back, assistance with repositioning in bed, or relocation of an external monitoring device. Teach her appropriate communication methods and reinforce their use.

- Help the patient use relaxation techniques to relieve pain. Also encourage her to relax physically between and during contractions as much as possible. Commend her efforts toward relaxation.

- Offer pharmacologic pain-relief methods as prescribed. Teach the patient about available choices for pain relief during labor.

- Administer analgesics as prescribed and as requested. Help prepare the patient for anesthesia administration as prescribed.

- Ensure that the patient receives support through each contraction as labor progresses. For the patient in transition labor without anesthesia, a support person should remain at the bedside to coach the patient through the increment, acme, and decrement of each contraction. Frequently reassure the patient about her success in managing contractions.

NURSING DIAGNOSIS

High risk for fluid volume deficit related to restricted oral intake, increased fluid loss during labor, and inadequate fluid intake

DESIRED PATIENT OUTCOME

The patient will maintain adequate fluid volume and electrolyte balance during labor and delivery

Outcome measurement criteria

☐ Blood pressure within normal range for the patient

☐ Skin warm to touch and without mottling or cyanosis

☐ Moist mucous membranes

☐ Urine output greater than or equal to 30 ml/hour

☐ Absence of ketones in urine

☐ Urine specific gravity between 1.003 and 1.030

☐ Electrolyte levels within normal ranges

Key interventions

- Monitor and document vital signs.

- Assess the condition of the mucous membranes. Provide oral care to moisten dry oral mucous membranes.

- Administer I.V. and oral fluids as prescribed.

- Report the results of such laboratory tests as hematocrit, urine specific gravity, and electrolyte and hemoglobin levels.

- Monitor and document fluid intake and output.

- Encourage the patient to void at least once every 2 hours.

- Notify the health care professional if ketonuria occurs.

- Encourage controlled breathing to decrease insensible fluid loss.

- Adjust the room temperature to increase the patient's comfort and decrease fluid loss through diaphoresis.

NURSING DIAGNOSIS

High risk for injury (maternal and fetal) related to complications of analgesia or anesthesia

DESIRED PATIENT OUTCOME

The patient and fetus will sustain no injuries from analgesia or anesthesia

Outcome measurement criteria

☐ Maternal blood pressure and pulse rate within normal ranges for the patient

☐ Absence of anaphylactic response to medications

☐ FHR within normal range

☐ Presence of fetal short-term variability and long-term variability in FHR

☐ Presence of FHR accelerations

☐ No nonreassuring FHR patterns

Key interventions

• Assess the patient for allergies and document them. Ask about her response to medications listed as allergens. Determine if the patient has received analgesics or anesthetics before. If so, inquire about her response to them.

• Assess and document maternal vital signs and FHR before analgesia or anesthesia administration.

• Continuously monitor the FHR pattern during and after medication administration.

• Administer a small dose of I.V. medication at the beginning of three to five consecutive contractions using the lowest port in the tubing. Discontinue administration and notify the health care professional if nonreassuring FHR patterns or fetal bradycardia occurs.

• Support the patient throughout epidural or spinal anesthesia. Also monitor maternal and fetal vital signs and document maternal and fetal responses to anesthesia.

• Observe closely for maternal hypotension. Be alert for maternal complaints of dizziness or nausea, which may signal hypotension. To expand circulating volume, administer a warmed bolus of I.V. fluid, such as lactated

Ringer's solution, or medication as prescribed. Reposition the patient in the left lateral position as needed.

- Monitor and document the fetal response to anesthesia or analgesia. If the fetal response is severe, administer a tocolytic agent as prescribed to inhibit labor.

- Observe for signs of anaphylaxis, such as dyspnea, cyanosis, and shock. Take or assist with emergency interventions as needed.

NURSING DIAGNOSIS

Ineffective individual coping related to ineffective breathing patterns, fatigue, fear, or lack of a support person

DESIRED PATIENT OUTCOME

The patient will demonstrate effective coping techniques during labor and delivery

Outcome measurement criteria

☐ Absence of hyperventilation

☐ Use of various effective breathing patterns

☐ Verbalization of the ability to continue labor

☐ Identification of specific concerns related to the outcome of labor

☐ Expression of an accurate understanding of personal and fetal status throughout labor

☐ Presence of a positive support person throughout labor

Key interventions

- Assess the patient's coping techniques during labor. Identify ineffective coping techniques and reinforce effective ones.

- Help the patient recognize ineffective breathing patterns, such as hyperventilation. Demonstrate various breathing patterns that she can use during contractions to promote adequate ventilatory exchange. Encourage the patient to control her breathing.

- Decrease the potential for fatigue by providing a restful environment. For example, organize nursing care to decrease the frequency of interruptions and encourage the patient to rest as much as possible during labor.

- Administer I.V. fluids as prescribed and offer high-carbohydrate juices and candies as prescribed to increase the blood glucose level and provide rapidly available energy.

- Encourage the patient and family to verbalize their fears and concerns about labor. Provide accurate information in response to their questions or concerns.

- Frequently inform the patient and family members of the patient's progress in labor and offer them frequent encouragement and reassurance. Help the patient and family recognize even small changes in effacement, dilation, and station of presenting part as significant changes.

- Acknowledge the importance of the support person. Reinforce the need for the continued presence of a positive support person for the patient. Relieve the support person as needed and remain with the patient in that person's absence, as needed.

NURSING DIAGNOSIS

High risk for low self-esteem related to loss of control of emotions and elimination

DESIRED PATIENT OUTCOME

The patient will express a positive self-concept in relation to labor and delivery

Outcome measurement criteria

☐ Absence of expressions of negative self-appraisal

☐ Absence of expressions of shame or guilt

☐ Verbalization of positive self-appraisal

☐ Acknowledgment of the unavoidability of loss of control of elimination functions

Key interventions

• Assess the patient's expectations for herself in coping with labor. Discuss her fears about loss of emotional control.

• Reassure the patient that she will receive support throughout labor. Discuss plans for a support person to attend the delivery. Involve the support person in discussing the patient's concerns.

• Encourage the patient to recognize that her behavior during delivery may not be similar to her normal level of control. Reinforce the acceptability of this lack of usual control.

• Inform the patient of the benefits of vocalization during the second stage of labor. Encourage her not to hesitate to use her voice while pushing. Explain that some women find it helpful to moan or grunt during pushing efforts.

• Assess for urinary bladder fullness. Help the patient void before the onset of the second stage of labor. If the patient cannot void, empty the bladder by sterile straight catheterization as ordered.

• Advise the patient that uncontrolled elimination is common during the second stage of labor. Reassure her that this is normal and that she should not try to avoid defecation because of the negative effects this would have on her pushing efforts.

Nursing Diagnosis

High risk for fluid volume deficit related to abnormal bleeding secondary to uterine changes during the fourth stage of labor

DESIRED PATIENT OUTCOME

The patient will maintain adequate circulating fluid volume through the fourth stage of labor

Outcome measurement criteria

☐ Blood pressure within normal range for the patient

☐ No narrowing pulse pressure

☐ Pulse rate of 60 to 90 beats/minute

☐ Skin warm to touch and without mottling or cyanosis

☐ Postpartal uterus firm and midline

☐ Absence of large clots in lochia

☐ Absence of spurting blood or continuous blood trickling from the vagina

☐ Urine output greater than or equal to 30 ml/hour

☐ Palpable peripheral pulses

☐ No confusion or loss of consciousness

Key interventions

- Frequently assess and document vital signs and the appearance of the patient's skin.

- While supporting the base of the uterus, frequently palpate the fundus to assess its firmness and position in the abdomen. Gently massage the fundus, if needed, to promote uterine contraction. Notify the health care professional if it is not sufficiently contracted.

- Anticipate finding the uterine fundus at least half-way between umbilicus and suprapubic area in the fourth stage of labor.

- Empty the patient's urinary bladder as ordered, if the fundus is not midline. Then reassess the location of the fundus.
- Document uterine involution for comparison with future evaluations.
- Assess the amount, color, and nature of lochia. Report bleeding that is heavier than one saturated pad per hour or spurting or continuous trickling of blood.
- Administer I.V. and oral fluids as prescribed.
- Administer oxytocic medications as prescribed.
- Assess and document the patient's level of consciousness.
- Monitor and document fluid intake and output.

NURSING DIAGNOSIS

Altered family processes related to the addition of a new family member

DESIRED PATIENT OUTCOME

The patient and family will begin adapting to changes in family functioning and will integrate the new family member in a positive manner

Outcome measurement criteria

☐ Expression of satisfaction with the infant shortly after delivery

☐ Engagement in initial bonding behaviors with the infant

☐ Demonstration of support and encouragement for the patient

Key interventions

- Promote initial bonding behaviors by providing time for the patient and family to be with, hold, and inspect the infant.

- Show the family members how to hold the infant in the en face position.

- Unwrap the infant momentarily and encourage the patient and family to inspect the infant fully. Point out unique features about the infant's appearance to promote their further investigation.

- Explain any characteristics of appearance that may have been caused by delivery, such as molding, caput succedaneum, or cephalhematoma.

- Assist with initiation of breast-feeding if the patient desires.

- Compliment the efforts of the patient and support person in successfully completing labor and delivery. Encourage other family members to recognize the patient's efforts.

- Be alert for early indications of lack of bonding or expressions of dissatisfaction with the infant. If needed, give the patient time to rest before engaging in bonding behaviors.

Manual extraction of the placenta

Manual delivery of a whole placenta or retained placental parts.

NURSING DIAGNOSIS

Pain related to the effects of manipulations used in manual extraction of the placenta

DESIRED PATIENT OUTCOME

The patient will experience little or no pain from manual extraction of the placenta

Outcome measurement criteria

- ☐ Absence of signs and symptoms of pain
- ☐ Report of tolerable pain

Key interventions

- Assess the patient's response to the treatment. Be alert for signs and symptoms of pain.
- Help the patient engage in diversional activities, such as controlled breathing or focusing on the infant during the treatment.
- Reassure and comfort the patient during the treatment.
- Administer pain medications as prescribed.

NURSING DIAGNOSIS

High risk for fluid volume deficit related to abnormal uterine bleeding caused by manual extraction of the placenta

DESIRED PATIENT OUTCOME

The patient will maintain adequate fluid volume and electrolyte balance

Outcome measurement criteria

☐ Vital signs within normal range

☐ Firm, midline postpartal uterine fundus

☐ Absence of heavy postpartal bleeding

☐ Absence of multiple clots in lochia

☐ Absence of uterine eversion

Key interventions

- Monitor and document the patient's vital signs during placental extraction and the recovery period at least every 15 minutes.

- Assess the amount and character of the lochia. Report bleeding heavier than one saturated pad in 2 to 3 hours or spurting blood.

- While supporting the base of the uterus, palpate the fundus to assess its firmness. Gently massage the fundus, if needed, to promote uterine contraction.

- Administer I.V. fluids as prescribed.

- Administer oxytocic medications as prescribed.

NURSING DIAGNOSIS

High risk for infection related to uterine exposure to pathogens during manual extraction of the placenta

DESIRED PATIENT OUTCOME

The patient will experience no postpartal uterine infection

Outcome measurement criteria

☐ Temperature at or below 100.4° F (38° C)

☐ Absence of tachycardia and tachypnea

☐ Uterine fundus nontender to palpation

☐ Absence of malodorous lochia

☐ Absence of purulent vaginal drainage

☐ White blood cell (WBC) count and erythrocyte sedimentation rate (ESR) within normal postpartal limits

Key interventions

• Assess and document vital signs, particularly noting signs of impending infection.

• Palpate the patient's uterine fundus to detect tenderness.

• Administer prophylactic antibiotics as prescribed. Teach the patient and family about benefits, adverse effects, and risks of these drugs.

• Assess the characteristics of the patient's lochia. Teach the patient and family to report heavy bleeding, malodorous drainage, or clots larger than a dime in the lochia.

• Monitor laboratory test results; report an increased WBC or decreased ESR to the health care professional.

Postdatism

Labor and delivery of an infant past 41 weeks' gestation.

NURSING DIAGNOSIS
High risk for injury (fetal) related to hypoxia secondary to decreased uteroplacental function

DESIRED PATIENT OUTCOME
The infant will display no injury from hypoxia during labor

Outcome measurement criteria
- ☐ Baseline fetal heart rate (FHR) of 120 to 160 beats/ minute
- ☐ Presence of average short-term variability (STV) and long-term variability (LTV) in FHR
- ☐ FHR accelerations with fetal movement
- ☐ FHR acceleration of 15 beats/minute for 15 seconds after scalp stimulation
- ☐ Absence of persistent variable or late decelerations
- ☐ Fetal scalp blood pH greater than 7.20
- ☐ Delivery of a viable infant

Key interventions
- Monitor the FHR pattern continually.
- Assess frequently for accurate placement of monitors on and in the patient. Document changes in monitor placement.

- Frequently assess and document maternal vital signs, maternal activity, baseline FHR, and periodic changes in FHR. Also document interventions, including medication administration.

- Assess and document STV and LTV. Anticipate decreased STV and LTV after analgesic or anesthetic administration.

- If STV or LTV are minimal to absent periodically, verify reassuring FHR pattern by performing scalp stimulation as needed.

- If variable decelerations persist, administer fluid by amnioinfusion as prescribed to cushion the umbilical cord against compression from contractions.

- Notify the health care professional of any suspicious, threatening, ominous, or chronic nonreassuring FHR patterns.

- If a nonreassuring FHR pattern occurs, prepare to initiate intrauterine resuscitation by repositioning the patient to improve maternal or uteroplacental circulation; discontinuing the oxytocin infusion to decrease the contractions' frequency, intensity, and duration; increasing the I.V. fluid infusion rate to increase maternal circulating volume; and administering oxygen by tight face mask at 8 to 10 liters/minute to increase oxygen flow across the placenta.

- Assist with fetal scalp blood sampling as ordered.

- Keep the patient and family informed about all procedures.

Precipitous labor and delivery

Labor that lasts less than 3 hours and delivery that occurs rapidly, possibly without appropriate attendants.

NURSING DIAGNOSIS

High risk for injury (maternal and fetal) related to the extreme force and increased frequency of uterine contractions secondary to precipitous labor

DESIRED PATIENT OUTCOME

The patient and fetus will complete the delivery without injury

Outcome measurement criteria

☐ Absence of signs and symptoms of amniotic fluid embolism

☐ Absence of signs and symptoms of uterine rupture

☐ Delivery of a viable infant

Key interventions

• Monitor and document the patient's vital signs.

• Assess the patient's perceptions of pain. Be alert for such statements as "Something's giving way" or "I can't catch my breath." Such statements may indicate uterine rupture or amniotic fluid embolism and require further assessment.

• Assess the fetal response to precipitous labor by using an electronic fetal monitoring device, if possible. Take measures to ensure fetal safety as ordered, including repositioning the patient, administering oxygen, and administering I.V. fluids and medications.

Nursing Diagnosis

High risk for altered fetal tissue perfusion related to inadequate uterine resting tone during precipitous labor

DESIRED PATIENT OUTCOME

The patient will maintain or exhibit restored uteroplacental circulation

Outcome measurement criteria

☐ Fetal heart rate (FHR) of 120 to 160 beats/minute

☐ Presence of average short-term variability and long-term variability in FHR

☐ No nonreassuring FHR patterns

☐ FHR accelerations with fetal movement

☐ Delivery of a viable infant

Key interventions

• Continually monitor and document the FHR, particularly noting decreased variability and nonreassuring periodic patterns.

• Report nonreassuring patterns or absence of variability to the health care professional.

• Notify appropriate additional health care team members to manage the precipitous delivery.

• Reposition the patient as needed to promote optimum uteroplacental circulation. Help her into a left-lateral (the most preferred), right-lateral, or knee-chest position, depending on fetal status.

• Administer oxygen at 8 to 10 liters/minute by tight face mask as prescribed.

• Administer I.V. fluids and tocolytic medications as prescribed.

NURSING DIAGNOSIS

High risk for infection related to lacerations of cervical, vaginal, perianal, or periurethral tissue during precipitous labor and delivery

DESIRED PATIENT OUTCOME

The patient will remain free of infection during the postpartal period

Outcome measurement criteria

☐ Oral temperature at or below 100.4° F (38° C)

☐ White blood cell (WBC) count within normal range

☐ Hematocrit and hemoglobin level within normal ranges

☐ Absence of extensive redness, edema, and warmth at laceration sites

☐ No signs or symptoms of urinary tract infection

☐ Absence of malodorous lochia

☐ Continued healing at laceration sites

Key interventions

• Monitor and document vital signs. Assess for signs and symptoms of systemic or local infection.

• Assess laceration sites for drainage, odor, poor approximation of edges, discoloration, and swelling.

• Assess and document the quantity, consistency, and odor of lochia.

• Evaluate laboratory test results and report abnormal values of hemoglobin, hematocrit, and WBC count.

• Maintain asepsis and strict hand-washing practices. Teach these practices to the patient and family members as indicated.

• Administer antibiotics and I.V. fluids as prescribed.

- Help the patient plan nutritional support of healing by including foods high in protein, such as chicken, fish, and legumes, and vitamin C, such as oranges, grapefruit, and strawberries.

NURSING DIAGNOSIS

Ineffective individual and family coping related to a panic reaction to precipitous labor and delivery

DESIRED PATIENT OUTCOME

The patient and family will cope effectively with precipitous labor and delivery

Outcome measurement criteria

☐ Expression of feelings about precipitous labor and delivery

☐ Acknowledgment of effective and ineffective coping techniques

☐ Use of effective coping techniques

☐ Adherence to health care regimen by patient and family

☐ Family participation in supportive care of patient

Key interventions

- Within the limits imposed by the imminent delivery, encourage the patient and family to express their feelings to one another and to the health care team members.

- Encourage the patient and family members to ask questions, if possible. Provide accurate information to help them deal with their fears and concerns.

- Help the patient and family identify effective and ineffective coping techniques. If necessary, teach appropriate coping techniques, such as communicating needs, and using simple relaxation, breathing, and pain-relief techniques.

- Assign specific roles or tasks to the patient and family members to involve everyone in a successful labor and delivery. For example, instruct the patient to signal when she feels a contraction begin, and instruct the support person to help the patient into a childbearing position, hold her legs, and encourage her while she pushes.

- Encourage the patient and family to communicate openly with one another and health care team members to discuss their feelings after the infant's birth.

Umbilical cord prolapse

Presence of a portion of the umbilical cord below or at the level of the fetal presenting part.

NURSING DIAGNOSIS

High risk for altered fetal tissue perfusion related to blood flow occlusion secondary to prolapsed umbilical cord

DESIRED PATIENT OUTCOME

The patient will maintain or exhibit restored circulation to the fetus that is sufficient to sustain fetal life until delivery

Outcome measurement criteria

☐ Relief of pressure on the prolapsed portion of the umbilical cord as evidenced by a fetal heart rate (FHR) of 120 to 160 beats/minute

☐ Presence of average short-term variability and long-term variability in FHR

☐ No nonreassuring FHR patterns

☐ FHR accelerations with fetal movement

☐ Maintenance of palpable pulse in prolapsed portion of cord

☐ Delivery of a viable, nonhypoxic infant

Key interventions

• Notify additional health care team members upon identification of umbilical cord prolapse, so that they can begin emergency interventions.

• Continually monitor and document the FHR. Be alert for decreased variability and nonreassuring periodic patterns.

- Reposition the patient to relieve pressure on the prolapsed cord. Assist the patient to a knee-chest or lateral position or place the bed in the Trendelenburg position as needed.

- Administer an amnioinfusion as prescribed for an occult prolapse.

- Attempt to relieve cord occlusion in a complete prolapse by maintaining steady counterpressure on the presenting part.

- Administer oxygen at 8 to 10 liters/minute via tight face mask as prescribed.

- Administer a tocolytic agent as prescribed.

- Assist with preparation for cesarean delivery as ordered.

NURSING DIAGNOSIS

Fear related to lack of knowledge about treatment for umbilical cord prolapse and its potential effects on fetal well-being

DESIRED PATIENT OUTCOME

The patient and family will display increased knowledge about treatment of umbilical cord prolapse and will cope effectively with their fears about its potential effects

Outcome measurement criteria

☐ Verbalization of accurate knowledge about the ominous effects of cord prolapse

☐ Acknowledgment of the need for treatment

☐ Acknowledgment and discussion of concerns

☐ Demonstration of appropriate affect

☐ Report of coping with fears and concerns

Key interventions

- Maintain a calm, professional demeanor at the bedside.
- Assess the patient's and family's emotional reaction to cord prolapse.
- Help the patient and family obtain accurate information about cord prolapse and the need for immediate treatment.
- Keep the patient and family informed about the fetal status throughout treatment.
- Encourage the patient and family to ask questions.
- Explain the rationales for treatments to the patient and family.

Uterine rupture

Spontaneous or traumatic tearing of uterine musculature.

NURSING DIAGNOSIS
Altered fetal tissue perfusion related to decreased placental circulation secondary to uterine rupture

DESIRED PATIENT OUTCOME
The patient will maintain sufficient placental circulation to sustain fetal life until delivery

Outcome measurement criteria
- ☐ Fetal heart rate (FHR) of 120 to 160 beats/minute
- ☐ Presence of average short-term variability and long-term variability in FHR
- ☐ No nonreassuring FHR patterns
- ☐ FHR accelerations with fetal movement
- ☐ Delivery of a viable infant

Key interventions
- Notify additional health care team members upon identification of uterine rupture and begin emergency interventions.
- Continually monitor and document the FHR. Be alert for decreased variability and nonreassuring periodic patterns.
- Reposition the patient as needed to promote optimum circulation through uteroplacental structures that remain intact. Assist her to the left-lateral, right-lateral, or knee-chest position, as appropriate.

- Administer oxygen at 8 to 10 liters/minute via tight face mask as prescribed.
- Assist with preparation for emergency cesarean delivery as ordered.

NURSING DIAGNOSIS

High risk for fluid volume deficit related to excessive blood loss secondary to concealed or apparent hemorrhage from uterine rupture

DESIRED PATIENT OUTCOME

The patient will maintain adequate fluid volume and electrolyte balance

Outcome measurement criteria

- ☐ Blood pressure within normal range for the patient
- ☐ No narrowing of pulse pressure
- ☐ Pulse rate of 60 to 90 beats/minute
- ☐ Strong peripheral pulses
- ☐ Skin warm to touch and without mottling or cyanosis
- ☐ No confusion or loss of consciousness
- ☐ Urine output greater than or equal to 30 ml/hour
- ☐ Electrolyte and blood component levels within normal ranges
- ☐ Coagulation study results within normal ranges
- ☐ Hemodynamic monitoring values within normal ranges

Key interventions

- Monitor and document vital signs and level of consciousness.
- Administer I.V. fluids, medications, and blood components as prescribed.

- Assist with evaluation of laboratory results. Report abnormal findings to the health care professional.

- Assist with insertion of internal monitoring devices as required.

- Monitor and document fluid intake and output and the patient's hemodynamic status.

- Initiate and assist with resuscitative efforts as indicated.

NURSING DIAGNOSIS

High risk for infection related to altered skin integrity and blood loss secondary to uterine rupture and cesarean delivery

DESIRED PATIENT OUTCOME

The patient will remain free of infection in the postoperative period

Outcome measurement criteria

☐ Oral temperature at or below 100.4° F (38° C)

☐ White blood cell (WBC) count within normal range

☐ Hematocrit, hemoglobin, and electrolyte levels within normal ranges

☐ Absence of localized redness, edema, and warmth at the surgical incision site and insertion sites for invasive devices

☐ No signs or symptoms of urinary tract infection

☐ Absence of foul-smelling surgical drainage

☐ Continued healing at the surgical incision site

Key interventions

- Monitor and document vital signs. Assess for signs and symptoms of systemic or local infection.

- Assess the surgical wound for drainage, odor, poor approximation of edges, discoloration, and swelling.

- Report abnormal WBC count and abnormal hematocrit, hemoglobin, and electrolyte levels as ordered.

- Maintain asepsis and strict hand-washing practices. Teach these practices to the patient and family members as indicated.

- Change contaminated dressings as ordered.

- Administer antibiotics, I.V. fluids, and blood products as prescribed.

- Help the patient plan for nutritional support of healing by increasing her intake of foods high in protein and vitamin C.

Vaginal birth after cesarean

Labor and vaginal delivery in a patient who previously experienced a cesarean delivery.

NURSING DIAGNOSIS
Fear related to labor and the potential for repeat cesarean delivery

DESIRED PATIENT OUTCOME
The patient will express decreased fear of labor and satisfaction with the plan of care

Outcome measurement criteria
- [ ] Verbalization of fears and concerns about labor and the risk of repeat cesarean delivery
- [ ] Expression of an accurate understanding of the anticipated course of labor
- [ ] Expression of accurate knowledge of the anticipated nursing actions during labor
- [ ] Report of satisfaction with the plan of care
- [ ] Communication of needs for assistance throughout labor

Key interventions
- Assess the patient's attitude toward labor and vaginal birth after cesarean (VBAC). Encourage her to express her expectations for this labor as opposed to previous experiences of labor.
- Determine the reason for the previous cesarean delivery and inspect for a lower uterine segment incision.

- Assess the patient's plans for anesthesia or analgesia use, various breathing techniques, pain-relief techniques, the support person's role, and desired positions for delivery. Incorporate the patient's wishes into the plan of care as much as possible.

- Reassure the patient about the safety of VBAC. Remind her that she will be monitored throughout labor for signs of danger to herself or the fetus.

- Briefly explain the use of the electronic fetal monitor and note that it will be used throughout labor.

- Reassure the patient that her comfort is important during labor. Discuss any limits on her free movement during labor.

- Briefly explain the rationales for administration of I.V. fluid or placement of a heparin lock for venous access in case cesarean delivery becomes necessary.

- Teach the patient about nursing actions during labor, including monitoring of contractions and the fetal heart rate, performing vaginal examinations, monitoring the patient's vital signs, and supporting the patient and family members.

- Encourage the patient to communicate her needs as labor progresses.

- Verify that the plans for labor management meet the patient's expectations. Modify the plan as needed to meet specific needs that she identifies during labor.

- Be alert for signs of lack of labor progress, abnormal vaginal bleeding, uterine rupture, or fetal distress. Immediately notify the health care professional if any of these occur.

Bottle-feeding

Infant feeding method that uses a bottle to administer prepared formula.

NURSING DIAGNOSIS

High risk for anxiety (parental) related to inexperience with bottle-feeding

DESIRED PATIENT OUTCOME

The parents will appear increasingly relaxed during feedings and will report increased confidence in their ability to bottle-feed

Outcome measurement criteria

☐ Absence of awkwardness when positioning self and infant for feeding

☐ Absence of comments expressing doubt about the ability to bottle-feed

☐ Expression of satisfaction with bottle-feeding

☐ Verbalization of the need to continue practicing bottle-feeding

☐ Contented appearance of infant after feeding

Key interventions

• Evaluate the parents' knowledge and experience with bottle-feeding.

• Explain that the first few episodes of bottle-feeding may seem awkward and more difficult than anticipated.

- Reassure the parents that feeding is a learned skill and success will be achieved through practice.

- Caution the parents not to misinterpret the infant's behavior. Initial difficulty with bottle-feeding should not be misconstrued as rejection by the infant.

- Teach the parents to use a comfortable position for bottle-feeding. Demonstrate the use of pillows for arm, neck, or back support.

- Administer an analgesic as prescribed and requested before bottle-feedings to promote the patient's comfort during feedings.

- Help position the infant comfortably for feedings, such as in the cradle-hold position.

- If the patient had a cesarean delivery, cover her surgical wound with a pillow before she positions the infant for feeding.

- Assist with initial feedings. Explain that the infant's sucking efforts may be weaker in the first 12 to 24 hours after delivery than they will be later.

- Help the parents recognize increasing success with bottle-feeding. Ask how they feel about feeding the infant.

- Encourage the parents to voice questions and concerns about feeding. Provide adequate time for answers.

NURSING DIAGNOSIS

High risk for ineffective infant feeding pattern related to inadequate knowledge of bottle-feeding techniques and practices

DESIRED PATIENT OUTCOME

The infant will display adequate nutrition, and the parents will demonstrate increased knowledge of appropriate bottle-feeding techniques and practices

Outcome measurement criteria

☐ Coordination of the infant's ability to suck, swallow, and breathe

☐ Verbalization by the parents of infant reflexes used in feeding

☐ Demonstration of proper infant positioning for bottle-feeding

☐ Demonstration of proper nipple placement in the infant's mouth

☐ Regular and sustained swallowing of formula by the infant

☐ Demonstration of vigorous sucking by the infant

☐ Description by the parents of appropriate hygiene for feeding utensils

☐ Verbalization by the parents of correct nipple hole size

☐ Demonstration by the parents of an understanding of feeding frequency, duration, and volume

☐ Demonstration by the parents of effective burping technique

☐ Verbalization of normal and abnormal regurgitation

Key interventions

• Assess and explain the importance of the infant's ability to coordinate sucking, swallowing, and breathing. For the infant who has difficulty coordinating these actions, recommend slow, frequent feedings with adequate breaks to allow for normal breathing. Reassure the parents that as the infant grows and practices eating, its ability to coordinate these actions will increase.

• Show the parents how to test the infant's sucking reflex by placing a clean finger in the infant's mouth to experience the power of the suck and tongue movements that promote feeding.

- Teach the parents how to elicit the infant's rooting reflex. Explain how this helps the infant turn toward the bottle.

- Explain and elicit the extrusion reflex, which causes the infant to stick out the tongue. Then show how to stimulate the middle to back of the tongue to elicit the sucking reflex.

- Inform the parents that stimulation on the front of the tongue causes apparent rejection of the stimulus. Advise them not to misinterpret this reflexive action as rejection of the formula.

- Describe the startle reflex, which occurs when the infant's head changes position suddenly. Encourage secure head support during feeding.

- Help the parents hold the infant in a close, secure position. Demonstrate the cradle-hold and en face positions while supporting the infant's head and back.

- Explain that the infant's head must be higher than its body during feeding to promote swallowing and decrease the risk of choking.

- Stress the importance of holding the infant's bottle—rather than propping it—to increase bonding and prevent positional otitis media, nursing bottle caries, and infant choking.

- Demonstrate how to correctly place the bottle nipple in the infant's mouth. The nipple should be on top of the tongue pointing directly at the back of the mouth, not at the tongue or palate.

- Show how to hold the bottle so the nipple is always full of fluid. The nipple should not be allowed to fill with air.

- Ask about the water source in the home. If water comes from a well or questionable source, teach the parents how to sterilize all reusable feeding utensils and use boiled water for formula. Explain that sterilization of utensils requires boiling them for 5 minutes (or using dishwasher sterilization) and allowing them to air dry. If water comes from a safe source, the parents can use tap water to mix infant formula.

• Caution the parents to avoid contaminating the nipple during bottle-feeding by touching it or allowing it to get dirty.

• Teach the parents how to evaluate the nipple's hole size. It should allow about one drop per second through an inverted bottle. A hole too small frustrates the infant; a hole too large leads to overfeeding and regurgitation.

• Encourage frequent feeding (every 2 hours maximum) during the first weeks as the infant demands. If weight gain is insufficient, tell the parents to awaken the infant for feeding after each 4 hours of sleep.

• Teach about formula intake. A neonate may consume 0.5 to 2 oz (15 to 60 ml) per feeding. After a few weeks, an infant usually takes 3 to 4 oz (90 to 120 ml) every 3 to 4 hours. An older infant may take about four 8-oz (240-ml) bottles every 3 to 4 hours during the day and may sleep longer at night.

• Encourage the parents to allow sufficient time during each feeding to relax and enjoy the infant.

• Teach how to burp the infant in the middle and at the end of each feeding, or more frequently if the infant has swallowed a large amount of air.

• Demonstrate burping positions with the infant on the shoulder and sitting with support in the lap. Encourage the parents to gently pat or stroke the back to produce a burp. Caution against overvigorous burping, which may lead to excessive regurgitation.

• Explain that infants normally regurgitate small amounts after or during feedings. Abnormal regurgitation occurs when the infant forcefully expels formula or expels a large quantity of formula between feedings.

- Reevaluate the parents' understanding of bottle-feeding during follow-up visits or phone calls. Reeducate as needed.

NURSING DIAGNOSIS

High risk for altered nutrition: more (or less) than body requirements, related to inadequate parental knowledge of the infant's nutritional needs

DESIRED PATIENT OUTCOME

The infant will gain approximately 1 oz (28 g) per day in the first 6 months of life and 0.5 oz (14 g) per day in the second 6 months of life

Outcome measurement criteria

☐ Identification by the parents of the infant's caloric needs

☐ Demonstration by the parents of the ability to calculate the infant's caloric needs

☐ Provision by the parents of a safe diet for the infant

☐ Appropriate caloric intake by the infant

☐ Absence of overfeeding or underfeeding

Key interventions

- Teach the parents that the infant should consume about 55 calories per pound per day and that most formulas provide 20 calories per ounce. Explain how to calculate the infant's caloric needs and the approximate number of ounces to satisfy those needs.

- Provide a chart that shows the average number of ounces required at different weights, but advise the parents not to interpret this guideline too rigidly. Infants demonstrate growth and appetite spurts—and increased calorie demands—at 6 to 10 days, 6 weeks, 3 months, and 4 to 6 months.

- Have the parents divide the recommended number of ounces evenly between feedings for a neonate. For an older infant, teach the parents to give more formula during the day because the infant may sleep longer during the night.

- Caution the parents to avoid overfeeding and underfeeding. Overfeeding can lead to obesity; underfeeding can cause dehydration and illness.

- Verify the parents' ability to obtain sufficient formula. Refer them to the Special Supplemental Food Program for Women, Infants, and Children (WIC) or other community resources as needed.

- Encourage the use of prepared formulas. Recommend avoidance of homemade formulas, which may not be nutritionally complete.

- Instruct the parents that formula may be moderately warm (not hot), tepid, or cool. To warm formula, they should place the bottle in warm water until the desired temperature is reached. They should not microwave formula because this results in unevenly heated formula that can burn the infant's mouth.

- Teach the parents to discard unused portions of a prepared bottle because it is considered contaminated.

- Teach the parents to note formula expiration times carefully. Some formulas must be used or discarded within 24 hours; others, within 72 hours.

- Encourage the parents to document the amount consumed by the infant, the amount discarded, and the feeding time to keep track of the infant's intake.

- Inform the parents of the recommendation to avoid using whole, low-fat, or skim cow's milk for the infant in its first year.

- Recommend that the parents not provide solid food or cereal for the first 4 to 6 months. After this time, on the recommendation of the health care professional, they slowly may add cereal, fruit, and juice to the diet.

- Weigh the infant at each visit and document findings. Based on findings, commend or reteach the parents as needed.

Breast-feeding

Infant feeding method that provides breast milk directly from the breast or from a bottle.

NURSING DIAGNOSIS

High risk for anxiety (maternal) related to inexperience with breast-feeding

DESIRED PATIENT OUTCOME

The patient will appear increasingly relaxed during feedings and will report increased self-confidence in her ability to breast-feed

Outcome measurement criteria

☐ Absence of complaints of shoulder, neck, or back pain

☐ Absence of awkwardness in positioning self and infant for feeding

☐ Absence of comments expressing doubt about the ability to breast-feed

☐ Verbalization of the need to continue practicing breast-feeding

☐ Verbalization of satisfaction with breast-feeding

Key interventions

• Evaluate the patient's knowledge and expectations of breast-feeding. If possible, provide general information and correct misconceptions before the infant's first feeding.

• Explain that the first few breast-feedings may seem unsatisfying. Reassure the patient that breast-feeding is a learned skill, that she can achieve success through practice, and that the infant will not suffer nutritionally if the first few breast-feedings are not highly successful.

- Caution the patient not to misinterpret the infant's behavior. Initial difficulty with breast-feeding should not be misconstrued as rejection by the infant.

- Teach the patient to use a comfortable position for breast-feeding. Demonstrate the use of pillows for arm, neck, or back support.

- Teach the patient to consciously relax her muscles while breast-feeding, which increases her comfort and enjoyment of breast-feeding and promotes milk flow.

- Administer an analgesic as prescribed and requested before feedings to promote patient comfort during feedings.

- Teach the patient how to position the infant properly for feeding. When she is comfortable with one position, demonstrate others that may be used when she is sitting or lying on her side.

- Recommend using the football hold position for breast-feeding after cesarean delivery to avoid pain at the surgical site. Alternately, cover the surgical site with a pillow before the patient positions the infant for feeding.

- Assist the patient to help the infant latch-on properly. Explain that the infant's sucking efforts may be weaker in the first 12 to 24 hours after delivery than in the future.

- Help the patient recognize increasing success with breast-feeding. Ask her to describe her feelings about it and commend all positive reports.

- Encourage the patient to ask questions and express concerns about breast-feeding. Provide adequate time for answers.

NURSING DIAGNOSIS

High risk for interrupted breast-feeding related to inadequate knowledge of the benefits of breast-feeding

DESIRED PATIENT OUTCOME

The patient will continue to breast-feed her infant and will demonstrate knowledge about the benefits of breast-feeding

Outcome measurement criteria

☐ Verbalization of the physiologic benefits of breast-feeding

☐ Verbalization of the psychosocial benefits of breast-feeding

Key interventions

• Evaluate the patient's understanding of the physiologic benefits of breast-feeding. As needed, teach her that colostrum supplies antibodies that provide passive immunity for the infant.

• Teach the patient that breast milk is easier to digest than formula; that it contains all the required fats, proteins, carbohydrates, vitamins, and minerals; and that its protein is less likely to cause allergic reactions. Also explain that breast-fed infants typically have fewer episodes of constipation or diarrhea.

• Teach the patient that uterine involution is stimulated by oxytocin production, which is triggered by the suckling infant.

• Discuss ways that breast-feeding promotes maternal-infant attachment by frequent skin-to-skin contact, en face positioning, and allowing the infant to focus on its mother's face.

NURSING DIAGNOSIS

High risk for ineffective breast-feeding related to inadequate knowledge of feeding techniques and practices

DESIRED PATIENT OUTCOME

The patient will breast-feed her infant effectively and will demonstrate knowledge of appropriate techniques and practices

Outcome measurement criteria

☐ Description of infant reflexes involved in feeding

☐ Use of appropriate hygiene practices

☐ Demonstration of appropriate techniques for positioning the infant, introducing the breast to the infant, avoiding nare obstruction by the breast, breaking the mouth-breast seal, and stimulating infant feeding

☐ Use of various positions for feeding

☐ Identification of effective latching-on

☐ Verification of emptied breasts after feedings

☐ Alternation of breast offered first at feedings

☐ Verbalization of recommended duration and frequency of feedings

☐ Identification of signs of a good feeding

☐ Eagerness of the infant to breast-feed

☐ Regular, sustained, and vigorous suckling at the breast

☐ Adequate infant weight gain

☐ Soft stools and more than six wet diapers per day

Key interventions

• Help the patient explore the infant's sucking reflex. Encourage her to place a clean finger in the infant's mouth to experience the strength of the sucking and the tongue movements that promote breast emptying.

- Teach the patient how to elicit the infant's rooting reflex. When the infant's mouth opens wide, tell her to direct the nipple into the back of the mouth, pull the infant in close, and watch for signs of proper latching-on.

- Help the patient identify signs of adequate latching-on: nipple tugging without pain, infant jaw gliding without chewing, breast movement without sliding of the nipple in and out of the infant's mouth, and pulling of most of the areola into the mouth.

- Explain and elicit the extrusion reflex, which causes the infant to stick out the tongue. Then show how to stimulate the middle to back of the tongue to elicit the sucking reflex.

- Explain that stimulation on the front of the tongue causes apparent rejection of the stimulus. Advise the patient not to misinterpret this reflexive action as rejection of breast milk.

- Describe the startle reflex, which occurs when the infant's head changes position suddenly and can cause biting. Encourage secure head support during and when discontinuing feeding to decrease the risk of nipple trauma.

- Reinforce the need for handwashing, breast cleanliness, and cleanliness of clothes touching the breasts to decrease the risk of breast infection. Teach the patient to change breast pads with each feeding and to keep the breasts as dry as possible.

- Instruct the patient to introduce the breast to the infant with her thumb on top and four fingers below it, which directs the nipple toward the back of the mouth. Encourage her to maintain this hand position throughout the feeding to support the breast and ensure emptying. Advise her to avoid scissors or cigarette holds when introducing the breast because they flatten the nipple and make latching-on difficult.

- Teach the patient about infant positioning for feeding. The infant's head, shoulders, and body should be aligned. The infant's and patient's anterior surfaces should touch in the cradle-hold and side-lying positions. The infant's side should not contact the front of the patient's body during breast-feeding.

- Instruct the patient how to use the cradle-hold position. Once in a comfortable position, she should roll the front of the infant's body toward the front of her body, tuck the infant's lower arm below her cradled arm, hold the infant's thigh or buttocks, and bring the infant to the breast. She should avoid bringing the breast to the infant.

- Explain how to use the football-hold position. The patient should place the infant on a pillow at her side, reach around and under the infant to support the back and head with her arm and hand, hold the infant's head level with the breast, and bring the infant to the breast.

- Describe how to use the side-lying position. The patient should place the infant facing her in bed, use a rolled towel or blanket to support the infant in a lateral recumbent position, and support the breast with her opposite hand. Caution her about breast-feeding a young infant in this position in a water bed or on a very soft mattress because of the risk of smothering the infant if the patient falls asleep.

- Teach the patient to check her breasts for adequate emptying after feeding by palpating the breast tissue. The breasts should feel notably softer; one breast may be emptier than the other.

- Reinforce the importance of alternating the breast offered first at feedings. Help the patient develop a way to remember which breast to offer first. For example, she can place a safety pin on the bra strap of the breast to be offered first, keep a chart, or offer the fuller breast.

- Demonstrate methods the patient should use to avoid obstructing the infant's nares during breast-feeding.

- Teach the patient to discontinue a feeding by gently inserting a clean finger into the side of the infant's mouth to break mouth-breast suction. This decreases the risk of nipple trauma.

- Advise the patient to feed the infant primarily on demand. Initially, this averages one feeding every 2 to 3 hours for 10 to 15 minutes per breast.

- Teach the patient to burp the infant when switching from one breast to the other, and demonstrate various burping positions. Explain that breast-fed infants typically do not burp as vigorously as bottle-fed infants because they do not ingest as much air.

- Demonstrate ways to stimulate an infant who falls asleep during a feeding, such as unwrapping the infant and providing verbal and tactile stimulation. Teach the patient that sucking is more vigorous at the beginning of a feeding or when the infant is well stimulated.

- Help the patient recognize signs of an effective feeding: 10 to 20 sucks in a burst, regular swallowing, milk let-down, breast softening, and infant relaxation and satiation.

NURSING DIAGNOSIS

High risk for interrupted breast-feeding related to cracked, sore, or inverted nipples, breast engorgement, mastitis, lack of social support, or separation from the infant

DESIRED PATIENT OUTCOME

The patient will continue breast-feeding her infant and will effectively manage difficulties that arise

Outcome measurement criteria

☐ Little or no nipple soreness

☐ Identification of techniques to avoid cracked nipples

☐ Absence of cracked nipples

☐ Demonstration of effective management of inverted nipples

☐ Appropriate management of breast engorgement

☐ Identification of signs and symptoms of mastitis

☐ Absence of mastitis

☐ Verbalization of feelings of adequate social support for continued breast-feeding

☐ Report of continued, satisfactory breast-feedings

☐ Adequate nutritional intake by the infant

☐ Demonstration of techniques for expression and storage of breast milk

Key interventions

- Assess the patient's breasts for blistering, fissures, and redness.

- Advise the patient that nipple soreness is common at first and that she can avoid continued nipple soreness by ensuring proper latching-on, infant positioning for feeding, and breaking of mouth-breast suction.

- Describe techniques to ease and prevent nipple soreness, such as expressing a small amount of milk before a feeding; using warm, moist soaks on her breasts for a few minutes before a feeding; applying ice to her nipples to produce numbness; beginning a feeding with the less sore breast and alternating breasts several times during a feeding; avoiding letting the infant sleep with the nipple in the mouth; and using ventilated nipple shells to decrease nipple irritation from bras or clothing.

- Teach the patient to avoid cracked nipples by altering positions for feeding and cleaning the breasts with water only to avoid soap's drying effects. Also suggest that she express a few drops of milk after feedings and rub them into the nipple to help soften and moisturize it. She should allow the breast milk to dry before covering the breast with a pad or bra.

- Stress the importance of maintaining dryness to avoid nipple cracking. Recommend frequent breast pad changes and the use of pads without a plastic layer because the plastic retains moisture.

- Teach the patient to dry her nipples by using a hair dryer on a low setting or briefly exposing her nipples to sunlight.

- Encourage the patient to maintain appropriate feeding frequency during episodes of nipple soreness.

- Promote feeding on demand to decrease the risk of breast engorgement. Explain that engorgement may occur 2 to 5 days after delivery and usually lasts less than 48 hours.

- Teach the patient to help her infant latch-on to an engorged breast by softening the breast before the feeding. To do this, she should apply warm, moist soaks to the breasts 10 to 15 minutes before feeding and express some milk by gently massaging from the base of the breasts forward until the areola is soft enough for the infant to grasp in the mouth.

- Teach the patient to use the same massage technique to hand-express milk during a shower or bath to decrease engorgement.

- Instruct the patient to wear a well-fitted, supportive bra at all times during engorgement and to avoid bras that are unduly restrictive, have underwires, or do not provide adequate support.

- Encourage the patient to take an analgesic as prescribed 20 to 30 minutes before feeding if she has sore or cracked nipples or breast engorgement.

- Teach the patient to identify and manage inverted nipples. Recommend rolling and pulling the nipple into shape before feeding, applying ice to the nipple a few minutes before feeding to increase nipple protrusion, using a breast pump shortly before a feeding to pull the nipple outward, or using specially designed breast shells between feedings.

- Encourage the patient to avoid using breast shields or artificial nipples for breast-feeding. Explain that these do not always promote nipple eversion, can inhibit milk production, and may confuse the infant.

- Teach the patient to avoid mastitis through good hygiene and prompt and aggressive treatment of sore or cracked nipples. Suggest eating a diet high in protein and vitamin C to promote healing.

- Provide written and verbal information about the flu-like signs and symptoms of mastitis: chills, fever, muscle aches, general malaise, and such breast changes as localized tenderness, redness, firmness, and heat.

- Advise the patient to notify the health care professional immediately if she develops flu-like complaints. Reassure her that mastitis usually can be managed easily and that breast-feeding does not have to be discontinued.

- Ask about the patient's sources of social support for breast-feeding, the feelings of the infant's father, and the breast-feeding experiences of family members and friends.

- Help the patient recognize the people who are likely to encourage her and those who are likely to discourage her from breast-feeding. Encourage her to seek encouragement from supportive people as needed.

- Refer the patient to community resources for breast-feeding, such as La Leche League, Resource Mothers, lactation consultants, and breast-feeding support groups.

- Reassess the patient's feelings and experiences with breast-feeding during follow-up visits and telephone calls.

- Teach the patient how to express and properly store breast milk when separation from the infant is anticipated.

NURSING DIAGNOSIS

High risk for situational low self-esteem related to inadequate milk production

DESIRED PATIENT OUTCOME

The patient will express satisfaction with her role as a breast-feeding mother

Outcome measurement criteria

☐ Report of fluid intake of 2 to 3 liters (2 to 3 quarts) per day

☐ Report of intake of 500 calories above needs before pregnancy

☐ Appropriate nutrient intake

☐ Report of feeling of fullness in breasts before feedings

☐ Report of let-down sensation at feedings

☐ Report of feeling of breast emptiness after feedings

☐ Soft stools and six to eight wet diapers daily from the infant

☐ Infant weight gain of 0.5 to 1 oz (14 to 28 g) per day in the first year of life

Key interventions

- Reassure the patient that inadequate milk supply usually can be managed effectively and does not reflect negatively on her maternal abilities.

- Explain supply-and-demand milk production: the more the infant suckles, the more milk is produced.

- Encourage the patient to consume 2 to 3 liters (2 to 3 quarts) of fluid daily. If needed, teach her to estimate the fluid volume of various drinking vessels and to record her daily intake until she establishes a routine for consuming the required daily amount.

- Recommend that the patient drink water, milk, or fruit juice each time the infant feeds. Urge her to avoid caffeinated beverages.

- Evaluate the patient's diet. Encourage her to consume 500 calories more than her prepregnancy requirement, usually a total of 2,500 to 3,000 calories. Provide caloric values of different foods to help her meet the caloric requirements.

- Encourage the patient to consume 65 g of protein per day and 1,200 mg of calcium per day. Refer her to a dietitian for counseling as needed.

- Before feedings, encourage the patient to assess her breasts, which should feel full and firm.

- Describe the let-down sensation and determine whether the patient has experienced it. To promote let-down, encourage her to use warm compresses before feedings and feed her infant in a quiet, restful, comfortable location.

- Teach the patient to palpate her breasts after feedings. At least one breast should be emptied at each feeding and should feel soft and pliable.

- Evaluate the patient's sleep and rest patterns. Explain that inadequate sleep can reduce milk production. Recommend that she get several naps or rest periods during the day.

- Evaluate the breast-feeding schedule, calculating feeding frequency from the beginning of one feeding to the beginning of the next. Recommend that the patient feed the infant every 1½ to 3 hours for 10 to 15 minutes per breast to increase milk production.

- Teach the patient to awaken an infant who sleeps longer than 3 hours and to stimulate the infant to a fully awake state before beginning the feeding.

- Encourage the patient to recognize daily soft stools and wet diapers as good signs. Multiple soft stools per day suggest proper nutrition; six to eight wet diapers per day suggest adequate hydration. If the infant does not have a stool for 2 days, advise the patient to notify the health care professional.

- Help the patient keep a record of the infant's weight. Encourage her not to weigh the infant daily so that she does not become discouraged if weight gain is not rapid. The infant who appears to be healthy and is eating well should be weighed no more often than every 2 to 3 days.

- Encourage the patient to use available resources for help with child care, housework, and meal preparation.

- Verify that the proper technique is used for breast-feeding. Observe placement of the infant at the breast, latching-on, sucking, and variation of positions for breast-feeding. Correct the technique as needed.

- Refer the patient to a support group or lactation consultant as indicated.

NURSING DIAGNOSIS

High risk for altered sexuality patterns related to ambivalence of the sexual partners secondary to lactation

DESIRED PATIENT OUTCOME

The patient and her partner will use mutually acceptable means of sexual expression

Outcome measurement criteria

- ☐ Identification of physiologic effects of delivery and lactation on sexuality
- ☐ Verbalization of common changes in sexual desire after delivery
- ☐ Report of satisfactory sexual expression
- ☐ Use of an appropriate contraceptive method

Key interventions

- Assess the concerns and beliefs of the patient and her partner about sexuality and breast-feeding, correcting misconceptions as needed. Explain that sexual activity does not have to stop because a woman is breast-feeding.

- Explain that decreased estrogen after delivery can lead to vaginal dryness. Recommend using a prescribed estrogen vaginal cream or water-soluble lubricant before vaginal penetration.

- Point out that orgasm stimulates oxytocin production, which stimulates the let-down reflex. Suggest that sexual activity occur shortly after breast-feeding when the breasts are empty.

- If the breasts leak during sexual activity, advise the patient to stop the milk flow by pressing firmly on the breast with the heel of her hand or wearing a bra during sexual activity.

- Point out that women commonly do not resume their previous level of sexual desire for many months after delivery.

- Inform the partner that women commonly do not feel desirable in the first months after delivery. Encourage the partner to be attentive to the patient's needs and help her feel more desirable.

- Reinforce the patient's need for adequate rest. Encourage the partner to help with daily chores so that she does not become overtired.

- Encourage the patient to reserve as much energy for her partner as possible. Reinforce the need for her to maintain an active role in their partnership.

- Encourage the patient and partner to make time for romance to promote satisfactory sexual activity. Teach them to allow adequate time for the excitement phase of lovemaking so that they are emotionally and physically prepared.

- Verify that the patient and partner do not plan to use breast-feeding for contraception. Tell them that pregnancy can occur the first time they have sex after delivery.

- Offer information about effective contraceptive methods for breast-feeding patients, including levonorgestrel (Norplant System), medroxyprogesterone acetate (Depo-Provera), and condoms with foam or vaginal inserts.

- Refer the patient and partner to sources for obtaining contraception, as needed.

Family adaptation to an ill infant

Process of incorporating a new, but ill infant into the family.

NURSING DIAGNOSIS
Grieving related to the loss of the idealized infant

DESIRED PATIENT OUTCOME
The patient and other family members will cope effectively with their grief associated with the infant's condition

Outcome measurement criteria
☐ Verbalization of feelings of grief and fear
☐ Demonstration of mutual support among family members
☐ Expression of an accurate understanding of the prognosis
☐ Use of appropriate support groups

Key interventions
- Help family members recognize that grief is an appropriate response to the loss of the idealized child.
- Encourage family members to express feelings. Deal openly with feelings of anger, fear, sadness, guilt, blame, frustration, and loss of self-esteem.
- Encourage family members not to become trapped in feelings of guilt, blame, or low self-esteem, which may hinder the grieving process.
- Discuss the stages of grief. Teach family members that reactions to loss have individual and cultural differences.

- Remind family members to support each other in their unique reactions to the situation.

- Help family members obtain accurate information about the infant's prognosis. Avoid offering false hope if recovery is unlikely.

- Be alert for inappropriate denial, which may indicate a dangerous lack of progress through the stages of grief.

- Help mobilize support among the extended family, friends, and religious community.

- Provide information about local and national support groups. Refer the family to clergy and other social services as needed.

NURSING DIAGNOSIS

Altered parenting related to the demands of caring for an ill infant

DESIRED PATIENT OUTCOME

The parents will manage parenting activities effectively and safely

Outcome measurement criteria

☐ Participation in planning infant care

☐ Demonstration of attachment behaviors

☐ Verbalization of knowledge of special care needs

☐ Demonstration of proficiency in infant care

Key interventions

- Keep the parents informed about the need for new decisions in infant care. Involve them in decision making about infant care. Support their participation in the decision-making process.

- Promote attachment between the parents and infant. Be accepting of the parents' abilities and inabilities as they learn to interact with their ill infant.

- Help the parents visit the infant soon after delivery. Give them photographs of the infant and promote frequent nursery visits.

- Encourage the parents to touch, caress, and hold their infant, if possible. Recognize that they may be afraid to touch the ill infant. Demonstrate safe methods of physical interaction.

- Encourage the parents to tape record their voices because the sound of their voices may be soothing to the infant. Use the tape when caring for the infant.

- Encourage the parents to bring clothing for the infant who can safely be dressed in such articles as hats, socks, and gowns.

- Help the parents obtain accurate information about the infant's condition and expected treatment and outcomes.

- Demonstrate how to feed the infant as appropriate. Support the parents in their newly learned skills.

- Support and encourage the patient's efforts to pump breast milk for the infant, if she desires.

- Provide time for the parents to be alone with the infant if possible.

- Help the parents interpret infant responses and recognize cues of satisfaction, overstimulation, and distress.

- Teach the parents how to bathe, clothe, position, and monitor the infant according to infant's individual needs. Support and encourage them as they learn new skills.

- Teach the parents infant cardiopulmonary resuscitation and management of an obstructed airway.

- Assist the parents in evaluating and altering their home as needed in preparation for their infant's discharge from the health care facility.

- Help the parents develop a plan for managing infant care at home. Encourage them to consider restructuring routine family tasks to incorporate the infant's needs into their daily lives.

- Encourage the parents to recognize that this is a stressful time for them. Urge them to support each other and verbalize their feelings openly and often.

- Refer the parents to appropriate agencies and groups for acquisition of needed equipment and social support. Encourage participation in support groups for families in similar circumstances.

- Provide emergency telephone numbers and a 24-hour number so that the parents can contact a nurse, if needed.

- Follow-up with telephone calls and home visits after discharge.

Family adaptation to a well infant

Process of incorporating a new infant into the family.

NURSING DIAGNOSIS

Family coping: potential for growth, related to the perceived need to learn infant care

DESIRED PATIENT OUTCOME

The family will learn to successfully care for the infant

Outcome measurement criteria

☐ Expression of realistic expectations for infant behavior and abilities

☐ Correct identification of the infant's physiologic needs and abilities

☐ Accurate interpretation of infant cues

☐ Participation in appropriate infant stimulation

☐ Demonstration of the ability to provide adequate food, warmth, rest, hygiene, and nurturing for the infant

☐ Verbalization of signs of infant health and illness

Key interventions

• Assess the family's knowledge of normal growth and development of an infant. Ask about their expectations of the infant's sleeping, eating, and social patterns. Correct misunderstandings, as needed.

• Teach family members that an infant may take weeks to establish eating and sleeping routines.

- Encourage family members not to impose undue time restrictions between feedings. An infant may need to be fed every 2 hours for the first few weeks of life.

- Explain that growth spurts and increased appetite typically occur around 6 to 10 days, 6 weeks, 3 months, and 4 to 6 months.

- Teach family members that infants commonly do not smile before age 6 weeks. Lack of smiling before this age should not be misconstrued as unhappiness, dissatisfaction, or rejection.

- Examine the infant in the family's presence. Elicit the infant's palmar and plantar grasp, rooting, sucking, extrusion, Moro, and Babinski reflexes. Explain that they are normal and enhance the infant's ability to feed properly.

- Explain the significance of the infant's physiologic findings: molding, caput succedaneum, cephalhematoma, lanugo, milia, vernix caseosa, acrocyanosis, mongolian spots, nevi, chemical conjunctivitis, subconjunctival hemorrhage, strabismus, normal heart rate and respiratory pattern, rounded abdomen, appearance of fontanels and genitalia, presence and appearance of umbilical cord, and flexed body position.

- Reinforce that infants are obligatory nose breathers and that the airway must be kept open at all times.

- Teach family members how to use a bulb syringe safely to remove the infant's nasal secretions. The bulb syringe should be depressed fully before insertion into the nose or mouth and should not be inserted too deeply. Pressure on the bulb should be released rapidly enough to withdraw mucus. The syringe can be emptied onto a nearby tissue before reinsertion into the nose or mouth.

- Inform family members that infants normally sneeze to clear the nasal passages; sneezing does not necessarily indicate disease.

- Teach umbilical cord care, as ordered, using alcohol at the base of the stump with each diaper change. Provide reassurance that the alcohol does not cause pain but may feel cold and cause the infant to cry.

- Teach family members that the umbilical cord stump probably will fall off within 2 weeks. Tell them not to pull on the cord to try to remove it prematurely. Demonstrate how to avoid cord irritation by folding the diaper below the cord.

- Teach family members to notify the health care professional if they detect signs of infection, such as purulent drainage or foul odor from the cord stump or inflammation of the surrounding skin.

- Advise family members to expect a few drops of blood when the umbilical cord comes off but to report more than a small amount of blood to the health care professional.

- Teach family members about the infant's immature thermoregulatory mechanism. Teach them to prevent heat loss by covering the infant with clothes and a light blanket when indoors and by using a head covering, as needed.

- Instruct family members about infant swaddling. Teach them to bring the infant's arms and legs to midline and snugly wrap its body in light blankets to provide warmth and a sense of security.

- Encourage family members to cuddle, caress, and stroke the infant. Explain that infants usually are soothed by gentle rocking or walking and disquieted by extreme or swift movements.

- Teach family members about the infant's sensory abilities. Assure the family that the infant will recognize them by their sound, smell, feel, and appearance.

- Encourage family members to use the en face position. Explain that infants can focus at a distance of 6 to 9 inches (15 to 22.5 cm) and that they prefer the visual stimulation of faces, geometric designs, and black and white objects.

- Teach family members that the infant will develop the ability to communicate needs through crying. Different cries may mean that the infant is hungry, tired, over-stimulated, understimulated, or bored. Until different cries develop, the family should ensure that the crying infant is fed, clean, dry, and warm and feels secure.

- Point out that the infant experiences a quiet-alert state every day and needs to interact. Encourage family members to use this time to engage in eye contact with the infant and to caress, cuddle, and talk to the infant.

- Reinforce the infant's need for frequent rest periods. Teach family members that infants commonly sleep 12 to 16 hours a day.

- Help family members recognize signs of overstimulation or tiredness in their infant, such as yawning, staring, irritability, and crying.

- Teach family members how to bathe the infant. Encourage them to keep the bath room warm and not to leave the infant exposed for long periods.

- Demonstrate an infant sponge bath. Using a soap-free cloth, gently clean the infant's face. With mild soap, clean the neck, head, upper body, and arms while leaving the lower portion of the infant covered. Rinse, dry, and clothe the upper body. Then expose and wash the infant's lower body with particular attention to the diaper area. Teach family members how to clean the perineal area thoroughly. Rinse, dry, and clothe the lower body.

- Discourage the use of powder, which can irritate dry skin and cause respiratory problems, and baby oil, which can clog pores and cause respiratory problems; encourage the use of lotion on dry infant skin and ointment only in diaper areas, as needed.

- Teach family members to bathe the infant daily and clean the perineal area thoroughly with each diaper change. For a female infant, they should gently separate the labia and wipe from front to back to remove irritants from the urinary meatus and vaginal orifice. For a male infant, they should clean the glans and shaft of the penis and the anterior and posterior scrotum.

- Demonstrate the proper technique for diapering, and have family members repeat the demonstration.

- Inform family members that the infant may receive tub baths after the cord stump falls off and the circumcision (if any) heals. Teach them to support the infant's head securely during bathing and to use only 2 to 3 inches (5 to 7.5 cm) of warm water. Caution them never to leave the infant alone in water.

- Discuss general aspects of infant wellness. Healthy infants usually sleep several hours a day, eat vigorously, have a lusty cry, have six to ten wet diapers per day, have a bowel movement about every day, and have periods of awake and alert states during which they are interested in interaction.

- Describe possible signs of infant illness, such as breathing difficulty, yellowish skin or eyes, lethargy or extreme restlessness, axillary temperature above 100.0° F (37.7° C), excessive mucus production, inability to be consoled, poor feeding, fewer than six wet diapers per day, and failure to gain weight.

- Evaluate family members' understandings of information provided and encourage them to ask questions. Provide a 24-hour telephone number to contact the health care professional.

NURSING DIAGNOSIS
Altered family processes related to infant care demands

DESIRED PATIENT OUTCOME
The family will adapt successfully to changes in family processes caused by the infant

Outcome measurement criteria
☐ Verbalization of feelings about changes caused by the new family member

☐ Demonstration of mutual support among family members

☐ Development of an equitable plan for managing household duties

☐ Use of external resources to meet family needs as indicated

☐ Expression of satisfaction with the infant

☐ Expression of satisfaction with themselves as infant care providers

☐ Participation in activities that focus on specific needs of individual family members

Key interventions
• Discuss the fact that although the birth of a child is usually a joyful family event, it also causes significant stress and requires much adaptation.

• Encourage family members to communicate openly and express feelings about changes in family functions. Explain that feelings of frustration are common and do not indicate poor parenting ability.

• Encourage family members to develop a plan for managing daily chores that allows the patient to obtain adequate rest and focus on her needs and those of the infant.

- Recommend that family members accept offers of help from support groups, including friends, relatives, religious groups, and community agencies.

- Assess family members' satisfaction with the infant.

- Encourage family members to commend each other for their successes in incorporating the new family member.

- Recommend that the parents take time, without the infant, to focus on their relationship.

- Encourage the parents to continue to spend time with each of their children to continue to recognize their place in the family.

- Refer the parents to social services, baby-sitting cooperatives, experienced parents, and counselors as needed.

NURSING DIAGNOSIS

Family coping: potential for growth, related to the perceived need to promote sibling adaptation

DESIRED PATIENT OUTCOME

The parents will successfully promote attachment between the siblings and the infant

Outcome measurement criteria

☐ Verbalization by the parents of the need for sibling attachment

☐ Participation by the siblings in early and frequent visits during hospitalization

☐ Demonstration by the parents of acceptance of the siblings' reactions to the infant

☐ Verbalization by the parents of the siblings' needs during adaptation

Key interventions

- Teach the parents to involve siblings in incorporating the infant into the family structure.

- Encourage the parents to allow siblings to visit the infant and their mother during hospitalization. Frequent visits can reassure the siblings that their mother is well, affirm the parents' love for them, and allow them to share in the excitement of seeing and holding the infant.

- Inform the parents that behavioral regression is common in siblings of any age and usually is short-lived.

- Encourage siblings to express their feelings about the infant. With the family, discuss the fact that the siblings' initial reactions to the infant may be less positive than desired.

- Help the parents accept that sibling adaptation is a process and that siblings adapt more easily when they are assured that their place in the family is not threatened by the infant.

- Encourage the parents to frequently reinforce each sibling's significance to the family, verbally, physically, and by spending time with each sibling individually.

Family adaptation to loss of an infant

Process of bereavement over the death of an infant.

NURSING DIAGNOSIS
High risk for dysfunctional grieving related to the death of an infant

DESIRED PATIENT OUTCOME
The patient and other family members will show signs of progress through the stages of grief and will express hope for the future

Outcome measurement criteria
- ☐ Verbalization of the impact of this loss on self and family
- ☐ Absence of continued denial
- ☐ Demonstration of appropriate affect
- ☐ Engagement in appropriate self-care activities
- ☐ Absence of severe, prolonged depression
- ☐ Use of external supports as needed

Key interventions
- Establish a therapeutic, trusting relationship with the patient and her family and validate their loss.
- Give family members time to hold and view their infant as appropriate; let them terminate the visit when they are ready.
- Discuss the stages of grief. Help family members recognize their current stage.

- Explain that progress through the stages of grief is not always unidirectional, noting that it is normal to experience multiple episodes of anger, denial, depression, and acceptance.

- Encourage family members to accept and recognize differences in individual and cultural responses to grief.

- Encourage family members to discuss feelings about their loss with health care team members and among themselves.

- Provide a lock of hair, footprints, handprints, blanket, shirt, identification band, and photographs of the infant as appropriate and as desired by the family. If they do not want to receive mementos of the infant at the time of hospitalization, store the items so that they may collect them later if they wish. Inform the family that the mementos will be kept.

- Teach the patient appropriate postpartal self-care measures. Allow time for the patient and her family to rest to promote emotional and physical recovery.

- Help the patient and family make decisions about care, including whether or not to remain in the maternity unit, having support people stay with the patient while hospitalized, naming the baby, and making funeral arrangements.

- Provide information about support groups, counselors, clergy, and hot lines for the patient and family. Encourage the use of these or other resources to help resolve grief.

NURSING DIAGNOSIS

High risk for ineffective family coping: disabling, related to the inability to resolve grief over the infant's death

DESIRED PATIENT OUTCOME
The patient and family will cope effectively with the loss of the infant

Outcome measurement criteria
☐ Absence of continued feelings of guilt or blame

☐ Absence of apathy

☐ Use of support systems

☐ Resumption of family activities

☐ Resumption of community involvement

Key interventions
- Provide accurate information about the cause of the infant's death, if known.

- Stress the need to avoid self-blame for the pregnancy outcome. Encourage the parents to recognize that blaming oneself or one's partner for the pregnancy outcome usually is inappropriate and does not help resolve grief.

- Teach family members the importance of open communication. Explain the risk of hurting feelings, misinterpreting meanings, and feeling frustrated if they do not maintain open communication.

- Help family members mobilize family support systems, as needed.

- Encourage family members to make decisions about removing or storing nursery items in their home. Reinforce that this is not a task that must be done immediately.

- Provide information about support groups for parents who have lost a child, such as Compassionate Friends. Encourage the parents' participation.

- Arrange follow-up care for the family through telephone calls and home visits.

- Assess the family's ability to participate in their usual activities of daily living.

- Refer family members as needed to a multidisciplinary team for follow-up.

Mastitis

Breast tissue inflammation, generally caused by Staphylococcus aureus.

NURSING DIAGNOSIS

High risk for interrupted breast-feeding related to pain, dissatisfaction with breast-feeding, and situational low self-esteem

DESIRED PATIENT OUTCOME

The patient will continue to breast-feed her infant and will report resolution of problems related to mastitis

Outcome measurement criteria

☐ Use of appropriate pharmacologic and nonpharmacologic pain-relief techniques

☐ Report of increased general comfort and decreased pain in affected breast areas

☐ Absence of signs of pain and infection

☐ Report of increased satisfaction with breast-feeding

☐ Report of self-confidence to manage further complications of breast-feeding

☐ Adequate nutritional intake by the infant

Key interventions

• Assess for signs and symptoms of pain and malaise.

• Assess for and document signs of infection, such as a temperature of 100.4° F (38° C) or greater, tachycardia, tachypnea, headache, nausea, and generalized muscle or joint aches.

- Assess the patient for cracked or inflamed nipples and redness, tenderness, hardness, and heat localized in the breast.

- Teach the patient to decrease pain by applying warm, moist compresses to the affected area before and between feedings.

- Teach the patient to gently massage the hardened area of her breast toward the nipple, as tolerated, before feeding to promote drainage of the area.

- Explain the appropriate use, benefits, and adverse effects of prescribed analgesics. Reassure the patient that the prescribed medication will not harm the infant.

- Encourage the patient to take the prescribed analgesic about 30 minutes before feeding for comfort if needed.

- Advise the patient to maintain bed rest for 24 to 48 hours after the onset of symptoms to decrease discomfort and promote healing. Explore infant care arrangements that permit this.

- Reassure the patient that the discomfort of mastitis should subside within 24 hours of beginning treatment.

- Inform the patient that during mastitis, breast-feeding is safe for the infant and promotes emptying of the affected breast.

- Reassure the patient that mastitis does not reflect negatively on her ability to nurture and breast-feed the infant.

- Provide information about resource and support groups for breast-feeding patients. Encourage their use.

- During follow-up visits and telephone calls, reassess the patient's satisfaction with breast-feeding and attitude toward continued breast-feeding.

NURSING DIAGNOSIS

High risk for ineffective management of therapeutic regimen related to inadequate knowledge about the medication regimen, self-care, and infant-feeding practices during mastitis

DESIRED PATIENT OUTCOME

The patient will effectively manage the medications, self-care, and infant feeding practices needed to cure mastitis

Outcome measurement criteria

- ☐ Use of antibiotics as prescribed
- ☐ Absence of increased oral temperature
- ☐ Report of fluid intake of at least 2 liters (2 quarts) per day
- ☐ Report of several rest periods per day
- ☐ Use of breast-feeding hygiene practices
- ☐ Absence or healing of cracked or inflamed nipples
- ☐ Use of proper technique to break the mouth-breast seal
- ☐ Demonstration of various positions for infant feeding
- ☐ Increase in feeding frequency to every 2 to 3 hours
- ☐ Increase in feeding duration to at least 10 to 15 minutes per breast per feeding
- ☐ Use of supportive but nonbinding bra
- ☐ Absence of breast abscess

Key interventions

- Teach the patient about the dosage, administration schedule, and adverse effects of antibiotics prescribed to manage mastitis.

- Reinforce the importance of completing the entire prescription. Explain that breast abscess may occur if mastitis is not resolved fully.

- Reassure the patient that the prescribed medication is safe for her breast-feeding infant but to notify the health care professional if the infant develops diarrhea.

- Teach the patient to take and record her oral temperature every 4 hours during the first 3 days of treatment and to call the health care professional if it does not drop within 12 to 16 hours of beginning treatment, or if it becomes elevated again within the first 3 days of treatment.

- Encourage the patient to consume at least eight 8-oz (240-ml) glasses of fluid daily. Recommend drinking water, milk, and fruit juices and avoiding fluids with diuretic properties or caffeine.

- Advise the patient to keep a daily log of fluids consumed so that she can effectively evaluate her fluid consumption.

- Stress the importance of bed rest for the first 24 to 48 hours of treatment. Help the patient mobilize the resources necessary to meet the needs of other family members during this period.

- Explain the importance of proper hygiene in decreasing the risk of further infection or reinfection. Teach the patient to wash her hands thoroughly before breast-feeding or handling her breasts.

- Recommend that the patient change breast pads after each feeding and change bras daily. Encourage her to keep her breasts clean and dry.

- Teach the patient techniques to manage or prevent cracked or inflamed nipples, such as expressing a small amount of milk before a feeding so that the infant does not have to suck as vigorously to produce let-down; using warm, moist soaks on her breasts for a few minutes before feeding to help stimulate let-down; applying ice to her nipples to produce numbness; starting a feeding on the less sore breast and alternating breasts several times during a feeding; not allowing the infant to sleep with the nipple in the mouth; and using ventilated nipple shells to decrease irritation of the nipple from bras or clothing.

- Teach the patient how to ensure latching-on and proper placement of the infant's mouth on the breast. Teach her to hold her breast with her thumb on top and fingers below to introduce the nipple to the infant's open mouth and to aim her nipple toward the back of the mouth.

- Teach the patient to break the seal of the infant's mouth on the breast by gently sliding her clean finger into the side of the mouth. Explain that this method decreases nipple trauma and can prevent inflammation. Have the patient demonstrate this technique and reinforce teaching as needed.

- Evaluate the patient's previous methods of breast-feeding. Watch for inadequate breast emptying, inappropriate positioning, and breast compression or engorgement.

- Teach the patient various positions for breast-feeding, including the cradle-hold, football hold, and lateral positions. Encourage her to feed the infant in her lap occasionally, leaning over the infant to ensure duct emptying. Explain the importance of using various positions for feeding to ensure adequate emptying of all milk ducts.

- Stress the importance of feeding the infant every 2 to 3 hours to help resolve mastitis. Instruct the patient to hand express milk or pump the breasts as needed to ensure complete breast emptying.

- Stress that feedings should last at least 10 minutes per breast to allow for adequate emptying. Teach the patient to palpate her breasts at the end of a feeding. Soft breasts are generally empty and firm breasts still have milk.

- Advise the patient to offer the unaffected breast first early in treatment, which ensures adequate let-down and can help empty the affected breast. As mastitis resolves, the patient should resume alternating the breast that is offered first.

- Evaluate the patient's bra. Teach her that her bra should be supportive but not binding and should not contain underwires. (Binding bras promote milk stasis and complications of mastitis.) Encourage the use of specially designed bras for breast-feeding.

- Teach the patient about the risk of developing breast abscess. Instruct her to notify the health care professional if tenderness persists or worsens, if redness spreads or does not resolve, if fever and general malaise do not resolve, or if the nipple displays a large amount of unusual drainage.

Postpartal common course

Typical physical and emotional adaptation that occurs during the postpartal period.

NURSING DIAGNOSIS

High risk for altered protection related to the effects of fluid loss

DESIRED PATIENT OUTCOME

The patient will remain free from injury due to the effects of fluid loss

Outcome measurement criteria

☐ Blood pressure consistent with prepregnancy baseline

☐ Pulse of 50 to 90 beats/minute

☐ Respirations of 16 to 24 breaths/minute

☐ Temperature at or below 100.4° F (38° C)

☐ Peripheral pulses of 2+

☐ Firm uterine fundus

☐ Uterine involution at appropriate rate

☐ Absence of postpartal hemorrhage

☐ Absence of orthostatic hypotension and syncope

☐ Fluid intake of 2 to 3 liters (2 to 3 quarts) per day

Key interventions

• In the immediate postpartal phase, assess the patient's blood pressure, pulse, respirations, uterine tone and involution, and bleeding every 15 minutes for the first hour, every 30 minutes for the next hour or until stable, every hour for the next 4 hours, and every 8 hours afterward. Assess the patient's temperature every hour until stable, then every 8 hours.

- Compare the patient's baseline blood pressure with the current blood pressure, particularly noting hypotension or pulse pressure narrowing, which may indicate hypovolemia.

- Be alert for tachypnea or dyspnea, which may indicate respiratory distress, and tachycardia, which may indicate hypovolemia or infection.

- Note an oral temperature above 100.4° F (38° C) in the first 24 hours after delivery; mild temperature elevation is common.

- Assess the patient's peripheral pulses and legs. Be alert for signs of venous thrombosis, such as decreasing pulses and areas of tenderness, redness, and heat on the legs.

- Report abnormal findings to the health care professional.

- Use the two-handed technique to assess the patient's fundus for firmness. Massage a boggy uterus.

- Note the location of the uterine fundus, which should be at or below the umbilicus in the immediate postpartal period, should rise to about the level of the umbilicus within the next 12 hours, and should involute by about 1 cm (⅜ inch), or 1 fingerbreadth, every day thereafter. At any time, a fundus that is palpated to the right or left of midline indicates a full urinary bladder.

- Administer oxytocic medication as prescribed.

- Explain to the patient the reason for uterine massage and the effects of oxytocin.

- Be alert for antepartal factors that may predispose the patient to postpartal hemorrhage: previous postpartal hemorrhage, pregnancy-induced hypertension, chorioamnionitis, anemia, previous bleeding disorders, hydramnios, multiple gestation, gestational diabetes, and grand multiparity.

- Be alert for intrapartal factors that may predispose the patient to postpartal hemorrhage: cesarean delivery, trauma from intrauterine fetal manipulations, mid-forceps delivery, forceps rotation of the fetus, vacuum extraction or forceps-assisted delivery, abruptio placentae, manual extraction of the placenta, prolonged or precipitous labor, labor augmentation or induction with oxytocin, magnesium sulfate treatment, or delivery of a large infant.

- Be alert for postpartal factors that may predispose the patient to postpartal hemorrhage: uterine atony, uterine subinvolution, or retained placental fragments.

- Assess the amount, color, and character of the patient's lochia every 15 minutes until stable. Consider saturation of a peripad in 1 hour to be heavy bleeding; a six-inch stain on a peripad in 1 hour, moderate bleeding. Weigh the peripads for a more accurate assessment of blood loss (1 g = 1 ml of fluid). Also position the patient on her side and check for blood pooling under her. Document the findings.

- Assess the lochia for clots larger than 2 cm (¾ inch) in diameter.

- Immediately report heavy bleeding, blood spurting, constant heavy trickling of blood flow, or multiple or large clots to the health care professional.

- Warn the patient not to try to get out of bed without assistance during the first 12 hours after delivery. Explain that the patient may feel light-headed on her first efforts at ambulation. Encourage her to change positions slowly to combat this feeling.

- Assist the patient to sit on the side of the bed for 2 minutes before attempting to stand and walk. Assess her blood pressure while she is sitting. Instruct her not to arise from bed if she is markedly hypotensive.

- Provide assistance for ambulation during the first 12 postpartal hours and longer if indicated.

- Teach the patient to use the emergency call light in the bathroom if she feels weak and light-headed when using the bathroom.

- Provide a shower chair for the patient to decrease the risk of injury while bathing.

- Explain postpartal diaphoresis to the patient. Reassure her that this is normal.

- Assess the need for linen changes in a diaphoretic patient to promote comfort and decrease chilling.

- Encourage the patient to combat the effects of hypo-volemia by consuming adequate amounts of fluid.

- Monitor fluid intake and output for the first 24 postpartal hours. Teach the patient and family to help document intake and output.

NURSING DIAGNOSIS

High risk for infection related to interruption of the first line of defense secondary to delivery

DESIRED PATIENT OUTCOME

The patient will display no signs of infection in the postpartal period

Outcome measurement criteria

☐ Temperature at or below 100.4° F (38° C)

☐ Absence of tachycardia, tachypnea, and hypotension

☐ White blood cell (WBC) count, hematocrit, and hemo-globin level within normal postpartal limits

☐ Absence of foul-smelling lochia

☐ Absence of purulent vaginal or surgical wound drainage

☐ Minimal redness, edema, ecchymosis, and drainage at sites of interrupted skin integrity

☐ Adequate approximation of wound edges at episiotomy, laceration, or surgical wound sites

☐ Soft, nontender abdomen

☐ Firm uterus with appropriate involution

☐ Appetite within normal limits

☐ Fluid output that approximates intake

Key interventions

• Assess and document the patient's temperature according to facility policy. Be alert for signs of infection, such as temperature above 100.4° F (38° C), excessively high fever, or temperature spikes.

• Assess and document the patient's heart rate, respiratory rate, and blood pressure. Note signs of infection or impending bacteremic shock, such as tachycardia, tachypnea, and hypotension.

• Monitor laboratory test results, watching for increasing or persistently high WBC count and persistently low hematocrit and hemoglobin level.

• Observe the color, quantity, consistency, and odor of lochia according to facility policy. Document findings.

• Note purulent drainage from the vagina, perineum, or surgical wound. Change peripads and reinforce or change abdominal dressings frequently to reduce the risk of bacterial growth on saturated pads or dressings.

- Teach the patient to change peripads at least every 4 hours while awake to prevent infection. Instruct her not to use tampons or douches in the postpartal period.

- Teach the patient how to perform proper perineal hygiene after voiding or defecating.

- Assess the perineum or surgical wound for redness, edema, and ecchymosis. Document and compare findings to previous evaluations.

- Assess approximation of perineal or abdominal wound edges. Document and compare findings to previous evaluations.

- Palpate the patient's abdomen at least every 8 hours, noting signs or reports of pain. Document areas of abdominal tenderness or rigidity.

- Palpate the uterus for tenderness and involution. Compare to previous findings to detect increased pain or subinvolution.

- Encourage the patient to void within 6 to 8 hours of delivery. Measure the voided amount for the first 24 postpartal hours.

- Ask the patient to void before routine postpartal physical assessments; then palpate for bladder fullness.

- Catheterize as ordered to remove and evaluate residual urine.

- Encourage the patient to attempt to void frequently and fully to prevent urine stasis and potential infection.

- Evaluate the patient's food intake. Encourage the patient to consume a diet high in protein and vitamin C to promote healing.

- Teach the patient about the therapeutic and adverse effects of the prescribed antibiotics.

- Notify the health care professional immediately of signs and symptoms of deterioration in the patient's condition.

NURSING DIAGNOSIS

Pain related to tissue trauma and the normal physiologic changes during the postpartal period

DESIRED PATIENT OUTCOME

The patient will report minimal pain in the postpartal period

Outcome measurement criteria

☐ Use of pharmacologic and nonpharmacologic pain-relief measures

☐ Absence of signs of pain

☐ Report of feeling adequately rested

☐ Report of decreased or absent pain

Key interventions

• Anticipate sources of pain, such as hemorrhoids, episiotomy, surgical incision, perineal edema, breast engorgement, breast-feeding, and back strain; take early measures to decrease the pain.

• Apply ice packs to the patient's edematous perineum.

• Use anesthetic sprays or pads as prescribed on hemorrhoids or the episiotomy site. Teach the patient how to use these medications properly.

• Administer analgesics as prescribed during the first 24 hours after delivery.

• Teach the patient about afterpains caused by uterine involution. Explain that multiparous patients usually experience more afterpains than primiparous patients.

• Help the patient communicate pain perception accurately. Ask her to rate the pain on a scale of 1 to 10 with 10 being the worst and 1 being the least.

- Observe for nonverbal indications of pain, such as grimaces, limited movement, guarding, and rapid, shallow breathing.

- Teach the patient the administration schedule, benefits, and adverse effects of the prescribed analgesics. If she is breast-feeding, discuss their safety for the infant.

- Teach the patient about the patient-controlled analgesia pump, if used.

- Encourage the breast-feeding patient to take an analgesic as prescribed before feeding the infant. Explain that breast-feeding stimulates oxytocin production, which causes uterine contractions.

- Explain that pain is easier to relieve if it is not allowed to become severe before intervention.

- Encourage the patient to request analgesics frequently enough to maintain control over the pain.

- Teach the patient about nonpharmacologic pain-relief methods, such as relaxation and deep-breathing exercises and sitz baths.

- Teach the patient with an episiotomy to squeeze her gluteal muscles together to decrease pain when sitting.

- Encourage the patient not to wipe her perineal area after voiding. Teach the patient to clean the perineum with a perineal squirt or spray bottle and to pat the area with tissue. Recommend remaining in the lithotomy position in the bed after voiding to promote drying of the perineum.

- Administer heat lamp treatments as prescribed for perineal pain. To ensure safety, place the heat source at least 24 inches (61 cm) from the patient's skin, make sure no linen comes in contact with the heat source, continue the treatment for no more than 15 minutes, and check on her frequently.

- Offer back rubs to promote relaxation. Change bed linens as needed to maintain a clean, dry bed.

- Help the patient take a bath if she desires. Place a folded towel in the bottom of the tub for her to sit on.

- Help the patient reposition herself in bed every 2 to 4 hours while awake. Provide pillows for support as needed.

- Tell the patient that adequate rest is essential for healing, and encourage her to rest frequently throughout the day.

- Limit visitors and decrease environmental stimuli if the patient requests.

- Reassure the patient that pain and discomfort will abate as she recovers from delivery.

- Assess the patient's bra. Encourage the use of a supportive, well-fitted bra to decrease the risk of breast engorgement.

- If breast engorgement occurs, apply ice packs to decrease the pain. Encourage the patient to avoid breast stimulation, for example, by directing the water spray in the shower away from her breasts.

- Reassure the patient that the pain of breast engorgement usually resolves within 24 hours.

- Administer analgesics to the patient about 30 minutes before planned interactions with the infant so that she is better able to enjoy the time with her infant.

- Reassess the patient periodically for consistency between reports of pain and rest and comfort.

NURSING DIAGNOSIS

Sleep pattern disturbance related to fatigue, facility routine, and infant care demands

DESIRED PATIENT OUTCOME

The patient will obtain sufficient sleep and will report feeling rested on awakening

Outcome measurement criteria

☐ Use of rest periods throughout the day

☐ Absence of reports of chronic tiredness

☐ Verbalization of the need to rest frequently throughout the day to meet infant care demands

☐ Report of restful sleep during the night

☐ Appearance of sleep on periodic assessment at night

Key interventions

• Explain the need for increased rest in the immediate postpartal period to let the body adjust to physiologic changes and to help her safely meet the infant's needs.

• Describe the typical schedule for postpartal care to the patient and her family. Help the patient plan for rest periods at times when she is least likely to be interrupted.

• Promote rest during the day by limiting visitors, telephone calls, and nursing actions during rest periods.

• Help the patient obtain sufficient sleep at night by providing a quiet atmosphere and reducing light, music, or other noise.

• Plan nursing care to avoid awakening the patient unnecessarily. Conduct physical assessments of the stable patient when she must be awakened for infant care.

• Offer relaxation measures before bedtime, such as a shower or bath, back rub, or relaxation exercises.

• Encourage the patient to notify a health care team member if she is having difficulty sleeping.

• Encourage the patient to continue planned rest periods at home. Recommend taking measures to protect her rest periods, such as taking the telephone off the hook or putting a sign on the door.

NURSING DIAGNOSIS

High risk for situational low self-esteem related to the discrepancy between the imagined and actual delivery, altered body image, and inexperience with infant care

DESIRED PATIENT OUTCOME

The patient will maintain a positive self-concept throughout the postpartal period

Outcome measurement criteria

☐ Report of satisfaction with the delivery

☐ Identification of common postpartal changes in physical appearance

☐ Report of realistic expectations for physical appearance in the first 2 postpartal months

☐ Recognition of the need for assistance with learning infant care

☐ Verbalization of satisfaction with progress in learning infant care

Key interventions

• Encourage the patient to discuss feelings about the delivery. Point out that most women imagine the delivery by the end of their pregnancy. Encourage her to discuss her imagined delivery.

• Help the patient compare her actual delivery to the imagined one. Encourage her to recognize that actual experiences almost never match the imagined ones.

• Be alert for undue dissatisfaction with the delivery. Encourage the patient to recognize the need to avoid blaming the infant for a delivery that did not fit her expectations.

- Assist the patient in examining her body. Teach her that abdominal swelling should resolve significantly in the first 4 days and that perineal edema and pain should resolve in the first week. Explain that her appearance will be more like her normal appearance by the end of the second postpartal month. Encourage the patient not to be discouraged by slow return toward her pre-pregnancy physical condition.

- Provide written information about postpartal exercises, and instruct the patient to resume exercise gradually.

- Encourage the patient to discuss feelings about her expertise in providing infant care. Point out that she may have a lot to learn about infant care and may feel awkward at first but that she will feel more proficient in time.

- Provide frequent praise and recognition for infant care activities performed by the patient.

NURSING DIAGNOSIS

Altered urinary elimination related to the effects of birth trauma on the urinary tract and to postpartal diuresis

DESIRED PATIENT OUTCOME

The patient will void without difficulty and will describe normal changes in urine elimination

Outcome measurement criteria

☐ Urine output greater than or equal to 150 ml at each voiding

☐ Less than 50 ml of residual urine after voiding

☐ Absence of palpable bladder distention

☐ Description of postpartal diuresis

☐ Identification of signs and symptoms of urinary tract infection (UTI)

Key interventions

- Assess the patient's risk of uterine distention. Note the time of delivery in relation to her last voiding, fluid intake, delivery method, type of anesthesia, and size of infant.

- Apply ice, as ordered, to the perineum immediately after delivery to decrease edema, which can interfere with voiding.

- Encourage the patient to void spontaneously within the first 6 to 8 hours after delivery. Measure output for the first 24 hours.

- Remind the patient to attempt to void every 2 to 4 hours while awake after her initial postpartal voiding. Encourage her not to delay voiding after she feels the urge.

- Promote voiding by helping the patient to the bathroom or bedside commode. Place her on a bedpan if she cannot ambulate.

- Stimulate voiding by running water in the sink, pouring warm water over the patient's perineum, or helping her sit in a sitz bath to void.

- Palpate for bladder distention at least every 4 hours until the patient establishes an effective voiding pattern.

- Teach the patient to rock slowly back and forth on the commode to promote complete bladder emptying.

- Monitor fluid intake and output. Teach the patient and her family to work with the health care team members to document her intake and output.

- Describe the normal postpartal fluid shift that causes diuresis. Explain that increased urination is not a sign of complications, but a sign of postpartal adaptation.

- Teach the patient to report signs and symptoms of UTI, such as burning on urination, inability to empty the bladder completely, bladder spasms, and difficulty initiating a urine stream.

NURSING DIAGNOSIS

High risk for constipation related to tissue trauma, hemorrhoids, and the normal physiologic changes during the postpartal period

DESIRED PATIENT OUTCOME

The patient will resume her normal bowel elimination pattern

Outcome measurement criteria

☐ Identification of physiologic factors that impair elimination after delivery

☐ Adoption of a diet that promotes bowel elimination

☐ Absence of painful defecation

☐ Absence of hard, dry stools

Key interventions

- Teach the patient about the postpartal physiologic changes that impair bowel elimination, such as perineal, anal, and episiotomy swelling; hemorrhoids; pain; intestine movement into a prepregnancy position; flatus; slowed peristalsis; and dehydration from labor.

- Inform the patient that a high-fiber diet and increased fluid intake promote bowel elimination. Encourage her to eat fresh fruit and vegetables, popcorn, and bran cereal and bread and to consume 2 to 3 liters (2 to 3 quarts) of fluid a day, including water and fruit juices. Recommend avoidance of caffeinated beverages, which tend to have a diuretic effect, drawing fluid from the GI tract.

- Administer stool softeners as prescribed.

- Advise the patient to pay attention to her body's signals and not to avoid bowel movements. Encourage her to use analgesics as needed before a bowel movement to minimize pain with defecation.

- Encourage the patient to avoid straining to have a stool.
- Provide a private, quiet place for the patient to meet her elimination needs.

NURSING DIAGNOSIS

High risk for altered parenting related to incisional pain from cesarean delivery and unmet expectations of labor and delivery

DESIRED PATIENT OUTCOME

The patient will exhibit a healthy relationship with the infant

Outcome measurement criteria

☐ Use of techniques to avoid incisional pain on physical contact with the infant

☐ Expression of satisfaction with the infant

☐ Participation in infant care

☐ Demonstration of nurturing behavior

Key interventions

- Assess the patient's interactions with her infant.
- Encourage her to express feelings about the delivery.
- Teach the patient to protect the wound site from stimulation by the infant's movement by covering her surgical wound with a pillow before holding the infant.
- Plan care so that the patient's interactions with the infant occur when the patient's pain is under control.
- Demonstrate infant care measures to the patient, as indicated.

- Demonstrate nurturing behavior, as indicated.
- Support the patient's efforts toward infant care and nurturing.

NURSING DIAGNOSIS

Impaired gas exchange related to shallow breathing and weak cough secondary to pain from the surgical incision

DESIRED PATIENT OUTCOME

The patient will maintain adequate respirations and gas exchange

Outcome measurement criteria

☐ Absence of cyanosis or skin mottling

☐ Respiratory rate of 12 to 20 breaths/minute

☐ Lung fields clear during auscultation

☐ No adventitious breath sounds

☐ Ability to breathe deeply at will and on command

☐ Ability to clear respiratory tract with coughing

☐ Use of splinting to promote deep coughing with minimal pain

☐ Arterial blood gas (ABG) and pulse oximetry values within normal ranges

☐ Tidal volume within normal range

Key interventions

- Assess and document skin color, respiratory rate, and lung sounds.
- Administer oxygen as prescribed.
- Encourage and assist the patient to turn in bed, breathe deeply, and cough every 2 to 4 hours postoperatively.

- Encourage and assist the patient to splint the abdominal incision with her hand or a pillow to decrease pain at the incision site.

- Evaluate ABG values and pulse oximetry and tidal volume measurements, as ordered.

NURSING DIAGNOSIS

Ineffective individual coping related to depression-induced inability to identify and express needs

DESIRED PATIENT OUTCOME

The patient will recognize and communicate her needs accurately throughout postpartal depression

Outcome measurement criteria

☐ Verbalization of an understanding that depression is common after delivery

☐ Recognition of the typical transient nature of postpartal depression

☐ Acceptance of self in altered emotional condition

☐ Participation in self-care to promote adequate nutrition and rest

Key interventions

- Teach the patient that postpartal depression (baby blues) affects about 80% of women after delivery. Emphasize that the condition is real—not imagined—and that it usually begins 2 to 3 days after delivery and resolves within 2 weeks.

- Encourage the patient to communicate her needs to her family. Explain that the family cannot anticipate all of her needs and that as her emotional state changes, she should attempt to communicate as clearly as possible.

- Teach the family to accept the patient's transitory depression. Reassure them that the condition is common.

- Encourage the patient to accept herself as her moods change or as she experiences bouts of crying or apathy. Teach her to remind herself that she will not always feel this way.

- Encourage the patient to do special things for herself, such as wearing pretty earrings, getting a manicure or pedicure, taking a warm bath, getting a back rub, listening to soothing music, or reading a new book.

- Explain that fatigue and inadequate nutrition may exacerbate depression. Encourage the patient to obtain adequate rest and nutrition to combat depression.

- Assist the family in planning ways to help the patient obtain adequate rest and nutrition.

Postpartal hemorrhage

Uterine blood loss greater than 500 ml within any 24-hour period after delivery.

NURSING DIAGNOSIS

Fluid volume deficit related to excessive blood loss secondary to postpartal hemorrhage

DESIRED PATIENT OUTCOME

The patient will display adequate circulating fluid volume

Outcome measurement criteria

☐ Blood pressure within normal limits
☐ Absence of narrowing of pulse pressure
☐ Pulse between 60 and 90 beats/minute
☐ Warm skin with no mottling or cyanosis
☐ Firm, midline uterus
☐ Measurable uterine involution
☐ Absence of heavy uterine bleeding or clots in lochia
☐ Urine output greater than or equal to 30 ml/hour
☐ Hematocrit and hemoglobin values within normal limits
☐ Peripheral pulses of 2+
☐ Absence of decreased level of consciousness (LOC)

Key interventions

• Place the patient in a supine position to promote blood circulation to vital organs.

- Assess the amount, color, and character of the patient's lochia every 15 minutes until stable. Consider saturation of a peripad in 1 hour to be heavy bleeding; a 6-inch (15-cm) stain on a peripad in 1 hour, moderate bleeding. Weigh the peripads for a more accurate assessment of blood loss (1 g = 1 ml of fluid). Also, position the patient on her side and check for blood pooling under her. Document the findings.

- Assess the lochia for clots larger than ¾ inch (2 cm) in diameter.

- Immediately report heavy bleeding, blood spurting, constant heavy trickling of blood flow, or multiple or large clots to the health care professional.

- Administer I.V. oxytocin (Pitocin) and fluids as prescribed to promote uterine involution and maintain circulating volume.

- Assess and document blood pressure and pulse and respiratory rates at least every 15 minutes until the patient is stable. Be alert for tachycardia or narrowing of pulse pressure, which may be signs of impending shock.

- Assess and document the temperature and appearance of the patient's skin.

- Assess the patient's capillary refill time.

- Assess and document the patient's LOC. Notify the health care professional of decreasing LOC.

- Assess the fundus for firmness and position in the abdomen. Gently massage the fundus to promote uterine contractions. Document uterine findings for comparison with future evaluations.

- Insert an indwelling catheter as ordered to prevent the bladder from displacing the uterus and to promote involution.

- Assess fluid intake and output and document totals hourly.

- Administer ergonovine maleate (Ergotrate Maleate) or methylergonovine maleate (Methergine) I.V. or I.M. as prescribed to treat persistent uterine atony or bleeding.

- Verify the availability of typed and cross-matched blood for replacement as prescribed.

- Administer blood as prescribed. Check the patient's vital signs every 5 minutes for the first 15 minutes, and then every 15 minutes throughout the remainder of the blood administration. Take her temperature every hour during blood administration and 1 hour after the infusion is complete.

- Assist the health care professional in checking for retained placental fragments as required.

- Report laboratory test results to the health care professional as indicated.

NURSING DIAGNOSIS

High risk for infection related to excessive blood loss and measures used to control postpartal hemorrhage

DESIRED PATIENT OUTCOME

The patient will display no signs of postpartal infection

Outcome measurement criteria

☐ Temperature less than or equal to 100.4° F (38° C)

☐ Absence of tachycardia, tachypnea, and hypotension

☐ White blood cell (WBC) count within normal postpartal limits

☐ Absence of foul-smelling lochia

☐ Absence of purulent vaginal or surgical wound drainage

☐ Minimal redness, edema, ecchymosis, and drainage at sites of interrupted skin integrity

☐ Adequate approximation of wound edges at episiotomy, laceration, or surgical wound sites

☐ Soft, nontender abdomen

☐ Firm uterus with appropriate involution

☐ Appetite within normal limits

☐ Oral fluid intake of at least 3 liters (3 quarts) per day

☐ Fluid output that approximates intake

☐ Absence of nausea and vomiting

Key interventions

- Assess and document the patient's temperature at least every 4 hours. Be alert for signs of infection, such as temperature above 100.4° F (38° C), excessively high fever, or temperature spikes.

- Assess and document the patient's heart rate, respiratory rate, and blood pressure. Note signs of infection or impending bacteremic shock, such as tachycardia, tachypnea, and hypotension.

- Monitor laboratory test results, watching for increasing or persistently high WBC count and persistently low hematocrit and hemoglobin values.

- Observe the color, quantity, consistency, and odor of lochia every 4 hours. Document findings.

- Note purulent drainage from the vagina, perineum, or surgical wound. Change peripads and reinforce or change abdominal dressings frequently to reduce the risk of bacterial growth on saturated pads or dressings.

- Teach the patient how to perform proper perineal hygiene after voiding or defecating.

- Assess the perineum and surgical wound for redness, edema, and ecchymosis. Document and compare findings to previous evaluations.

- Assess approximation of perineal or abdominal wound edges. Document and compare findings to previous evaluations.

- Assist with opening wounds as needed to facilitate drainage. Irrigate and pack open wounds as ordered.

- Palpate the patient's abdomen at least every 4 hours, noting signs and reports of pain. Document areas of abdominal tenderness or rigidity.

- Palpate the uterus for tenderness and involution. Compare findings to previous evaluations to detect increased pain or subinvolution.

- Evaluate the patient's food intake. Encourage her to consume a diet high in protein and vitamin C to promote healing.

- Monitor fluid intake and output. Teach the patient and her family how to measure and assist with documenting it.

- Evaluate daily fluid intake and output, adding estimates of insensible fluid loss and fluid loss by vomiting to the totals.

- When the patient can tolerate oral intake, force fluids as needed to increase her intake to at least 3 liters (3 quarts) per day.

- Assess the patient for nausea and vomiting, which may indicate sepsis and paralytic ileus.

- Administer antiemetics as prescribed. Assess bowel sounds at least every 4 hours to detect paralytic ileus and other complications.

- Use low suction on a nasogastric tube as ordered to decompress the bowel.

- Obtain specimens for culture and sensitivity testing as ordered. Report test results to the health care professional.

- Teach the patient about the benefits and adverse effects of I.V. antibiotics.
- Notify the health care professional immediately of signs and symptoms of deterioration in the patient's condition.

NURSING DIAGNOSIS

High risk for altered parenting related to delayed attachment secondary to hemorrhage-induced fatigue

DESIRED PATIENT OUTCOME

The patient will demonstrate appropriate parenting and attachment behaviors within the limitations imposed by postpartal hemorrhage

Outcome measurement criteria

☐ Acknowledgment of the need for increased rest periods

☐ Description of the limited duration of the need for increased rest

☐ Verbalization of satisfaction with the infant

☐ Participation in decision making about infant care

☐ Participation in infant care as possible

☐ Demonstration of nurturing behavior

Key interventions

- Assess the patient's reaction to the infant. Encourage her to express feelings about the delivery.
- Be alert for statements indicating negative feelings toward the infant. Explain the causes of postpartal hemorrhage, and encourage the patient not to blame the infant for her condition.
- Explain the need for increased rest periods to promote recovery.

- Reassure the patient that the infant's needs are being met; encourage her to accept the need to allow others to provide infant care at this time.

- Emphasize that the patient should feel more satisfied with providing infant care when she has recovered from fatigue.

- Explain that the need for separation is only temporary.

- Involve the patient in planning for her infant's care as much as she desires.

- Provide photographs of the infant for the patient to keep at the bedside.

- Encourage health care team members and family members who are providing infant care to give reports to the patient about the infant.

- Praise the patient's efforts to rest and recover from fatigue.

Postpartal infections

Pathogen invasion and excessive growth in the fetal mem-
branes and amniotic fluid (chorioamnionitis), reproductive
tract, or surgical wound created for cesarean delivery.

NURSING DIAGNOSIS
High risk for infection (postpartal) related to
chorioamnionitis

DESIRED PATIENT OUTCOME
The patient will remain free of infection during the postpartal period

Outcome measurement criteria
☐ Oral temperature at or below 100.4° F (38° C)
☐ No tachycardia or tachypnea
☐ Laboratory values within normal limits
☐ Absence of severe uterine tenderness
☐ Absence of foul-smelling lochia
☐ Absence of foul-smelling drainage from the episiotomy
site or surgical wound

Key interventions
• Monitor and document vital signs. Be alert for increasing temperature, pulse rate, and respiratory rate.
• Assist with evaluating and reporting results of ordered
laboratory tests, including complete blood count (CBC)
with differential, hemoglobin, and hematocrit. Be alert
for increasing white blood cell (WBC) count, decreasing
red blood cell count, and decreasing erythrocyte sedimentation rate.

- Assess and document the patient's ability to tolerate uterine palpation.

- Assess and document the amount and character of lochia.

- Assess the amount and character of drainage from the episiotomy site or surgical wound.

- Administer oral fluids, I.V. fluids, and antibiotics as prescribed. Teach the patient about the benefits, risks, and adverse effects of all prescribed medications.

- Assist with planning nutritional support of healing. Encourage the patient to select foods high in protein and vitamin C to promote healing.

NURSING DIAGNOSIS

High risk for fluid volume deficit related to excessive uterine bleeding secondary to chorioamnionitis-induced uterine atony

DESIRED PATIENT OUTCOME

The patient will maintain adequate fluid volume and electrolyte balance

Outcome measurement criteria

☐ Blood pressure within normal range for the patient

☐ Absence of narrowing pulse pressure

☐ Pulse rate of 60 to 90 beats/minute

☐ Skin warm to touch without mottling or cyanosis

☐ Firm, midline uterus with appropriate involution

☐ Absence of heavy postpartal bleeding

☐ Absence of large clots in lochia

☐ Urine output greater than or equal to 30 ml/hour

☐ Hematocrit, hemoglobin, CBC, and electrolyte values within normal ranges

☐ Strong peripheral pulses

☐ No confusion or loss of consciousness

Key interventions

• Monitor and document vital signs and skin appearance.

• Assess the amount and character of lochia. Report bleeding heavier than one saturated pad in 2 to 3 hours or a spurting blood flow.

• While supporting the base of the uterus, assess the fundus for firmness and position in the abdomen. Gently massage the fundus if necessary to promote uterine contractions.

• Document uterine status for comparison with future evaluations.

• Administer I.V. and oral fluids as prescribed.

• Administer oxytocin (Pitocin) as prescribed.

• Assess and document the patient's level of consciousness.

• Compare laboratory results with previous reports. Report abnormal laboratory values related to fluid volume and electrolyte balance.

• Monitor and document fluid intake and output.

NURSING DIAGNOSIS

High risk for injury related to possible bacteremic shock secondary to a postpartal infection

DESIRED PATIENT OUTCOME

The patient will remain free from injury caused by uncontrolled infection

Outcome measurement criteria

- ☐ Temperature of 100.4° F (38° C) or less
- ☐ Absence of tachycardia, tachypnea, and hypotension
- ☐ WBC count within normal limits
- ☐ Absence of foul-smelling lochia
- ☐ Absence of purulent vaginal or surgical wound drainage
- ☐ Decreased redness, edema, ecchymosis, and drainage at sites of interrupted skin integrity
- ☐ Adequate approximation of wound edges at episiotomy, laceration, or surgical wound sites
- ☐ Soft, nontender abdomen
- ☐ Firm uterus with appropriate involution
- ☐ Appetite within normal limits
- ☐ Oral fluid intake of at least 3 liters (3 quarts) per day
- ☐ Fluid output that approximates intake
- ☐ Absence of nausea and vomiting

Key interventions

- Assess and document the patient's temperature at least every 4 hours. Be alert for signs of infection, such as temperature above 100.4° F (38° C), excessively high fever, or temperature spikes.
- Assess and document the patient's heart rate, respiratory rate, and blood pressure. Note signs of infection or impending bacteremic shock, such as tachycardia, tachypnea, and hypotension.
- Review laboratory test results, watching for increasing or persistently high WBC count.
- Observe the color, quantity, consistency, and odor of lochia every 4 hours. Document findings.

- Note purulent drainage from the vagina, perineum, or surgical wound. Change peripads and reinforce or change abdominal dressings frequently to reduce the risk of bacterial growth on saturated pads or dressings.

- Teach the patient how to perform proper perineal hygiene after voiding or defecating. For example, show her how to use a squirt or spray bottle after voiding and pat the rinsed area with tissue.

- Assess the perineum and surgical wound for redness, edema, and ecchymosis. Document and compare findings to previous evaluations.

- Assess approximation of perineal or abdominal wound edges. Document and compare findings to previous evaluations.

- Assist with opening wounds as needed to facilitate drainage. Irrigate and pack open wounds as ordered.

- Palpate the patient's abdomen at least every 4 hours, noting signs and reports of pain. Document areas of abdominal tenderness or rigidity.

- Palpate the uterus for tenderness and involution. Compare findings to previous evaluations to detect increased pain or subinvolution.

- Evaluate the patient's food intake. Encourage her to consume a diet high in protein and vitamin C to promote healing.

- Monitor fluid intake and output. Teach the patient and her family how to measure and assist with documenting it.

- Evaluate daily fluid intake and output, adding estimates of insensible fluid loss and fluid loss by vomiting to the totals.

- When the patient can tolerate oral intake, force fluids as needed to increase her intake to at least 3 liters (3 quarts) per day.

- Assess the patient for nausea and vomiting, which may indicate sepsis and paralytic ileus.

- Administer antiemetics as prescribed. Assess bowel sounds at least every 4 hours to detect paralytic ileus and other complications.

- Use low suction on a nasogastric tube as ordered to decompress the bowel.

- Obtain specimens for culture and sensitivity testing as ordered. Report test results to the health care professional.

- Administer I.V. antibiotics as prescribed, and teach the patient about their benefits and adverse effects.

- Notify the health care professional immediately of signs and symptoms of deterioration in the patient's condition.

NURSING DIAGNOSIS
Pain related to the effects of infection

DESIRED PATIENT OUTCOME
The patient will report relief from pain

Outcome measurement criteria
☐ Absence of signs and reports of pain
☐ Use of pharmacologic and nonpharmacologic pain-relief measures
☐ Report of feeling adequately rested
☐ Verbalization of increased comfort

Key interventions
- Help the patient to communicate pain perception accurately. Ask her to rate the pain on a scale of 1 to 10, with 10 being the worst and 1 being the least.

- Observe for nonverbal indications of pain, such as grimaces, limited movement, guarding, and rapid or shallow breathing.

- Teach the patient the administration schedule, benefits, and adverse effects of prescribed analgesics and antipyretics. For a breast-feeding patient, also discuss their safe use during breast-feeding. If breast-feeding must be interrupted because of medication use, show the patient how to use a breast pump to continue milk production until breast-feeding can resume.

- Explain that pain is easier to relieve if it does not become severe before intervention. Encourage the patient to request analgesics frequently enough to control the pain.

- Teach the patient about nonpharmacologic pain-relief measures, such as relaxation and deep-breathing exercises and the use of ice packs or heating pads on painful areas.

- Offer back rubs to promote relaxation. Change bed linens frequently for the patient who is diaphoretic.

- Help the patient reposition herself in the bed every 2 to 4 hours. Provide pillows for support as needed.

- Teach the patient that adequate rest promotes healing. To promote rest, limit visitors and decrease environmental stimuli.

- Reassure the patient that her pain and discomfort will subside as her infection resolves.

NURSING DIAGNOSIS

High risk for altered parenting related to delayed attachment secondary to malaise and forced separation from the infant

DESIRED PATIENT OUTCOME

The patient will demonstrate appropriate parenting and attachment behaviors within limitations imposed by the infection

Outcome measurement criteria

☐ Acknowledgment of the need for forced separation

☐ Verbalization of the limited duration of forced separation

☐ Report of satisfaction with the infant

☐ Participation in decision making about infant care

☐ Participation in as much infant care as possible

☐ Demonstration of nurturing behavior

Key interventions

• Assess the patient's reaction to the infant. Encourage her to express feelings about the delivery and forced separation.

• Be alert for statements indicating negative feelings toward the infant. Explain the causes of postpartal infection, and encourage the patient not to blame the infant for her condition.

• Reinforce the need for separation from the infant to decrease the risk of infection transmission. Explain that the need for separation is only temporary.

• Involve the patient in planning for her infant's care as much as she desires.

• Teach or reinforce knowledge of infant care. Have the patient practice with a doll as appropriate.

• Encourage the patient to visit the nursery when she is able so that she can see her infant. Provide photographs of the infant for her to keep at the bedside.

• Support her efforts at infant care and nurturing.

Pulmonary embolus

Obstruction of blood flow through the pulmonary vessel caused by a clot that was moved by the blood from another part of the body.

NURSING DIAGNOSIS

High risk for inability to sustain spontaneous ventilation related to compromised cardiopulmonary status secondary to pulmonary embolus

DESIRED PATIENT OUTCOME

The patient will resume normal respiratory patterns

Outcome measurement criteria

☐ Respiratory rate of 12 to 20 breaths/minute

☐ Clear lungs on auscultation

☐ Absence of dyspnea, restlessness, and apprehension

☐ Absence of accessory muscle use for breathing

☐ Ability to clear mucus and fluid from respiratory tract

☐ Tidal volume within normal limits

☐ Arterial blood gas (ABG) values within normal limits

☐ Absence of decreased level of consciousness (LOC)

Key interventions

• Frequently assess and document the patient's respiratory status.

• Be alert for signs of respiratory distress, such as dyspnea, tachypnea, increased apprehension and restlessness, accessory muscle use for breathing, and pleural friction rub.

- Administer oxygen as prescribed at 1 to 2 liters per minute by nasal prongs.

- As prescribed, administer morphine sulfate (Astramorph) I.V. to decrease the oxygen demand; aqueous theophylline I.V. to dilate the bronchi; digoxin (Lanoxin) I.V. to decrease oxygen demand and control arrhythmias; and fibrinolytic drugs I.V. to dissolve clots.

- Assess the availability of typed and cross-matched packed red blood cells and fresh frozen plasma as prescribed.

- Review ABG analysis or pulse oximetry results as ordered, particularly noting increasing hypoxia and reporting significant findings.

- Assess and document the patient's LOC.

- Reposition the patient as needed to promote ventilation.

- Assess and document the patient's ability to clear her respiratory tract. Suction the respiratory tract as needed.

- Assist with intubation as ordered.

- Initiate or assist with resuscitative efforts as required.

NURSING DIAGNOSIS

Fear related to lack of knowledge about the disorder's treatment and potential effects

DESIRED PATIENT OUTCOME

The patient and family will demonstrate increased knowledge about pulmonary embolus treatments and will report tolerance of feelings about the disorder's potential effects

Outcome measurement criteria

☐ Verbalization of accurate knowledge about the disorder

☐ Verbalization of the need for treatment

☐ Acknowledgment and discussion of concerns

☐ Demonstration of appropriate range of feelings

Key interventions

• Maintain a calm, professional behavior at the bedside and with family members. Use clear, concise statements to communicate with the patient and family.

• Help the patient and family gain accurate information about pulmonary embolus and the need for treatment.

• Within the limits imposed by emergency or resuscitative efforts, explain procedures to the patient and family.

• Help the patient and family identify and use resources to promote discussion of feelings, such as other family members, other health care team members, and clergy members.

• Assess the patient and family members for persistent flat affect, which may signal ineffective coping or shock.

Urinary bladder distention

*Incomplete emptying and excessive residual urine that causes
overdistention of the bladder.*

NURSING DIAGNOSIS

Altered urinary elimination related to urine stasis secondary to mechanical trauma of the urinary tract, the effects
of anesthesia, altered voiding reflex, postpartal diuresis, or
bladder atony

DESIRED PATIENT OUTCOME

The patient will resume normal urinary elimination
patterns

Outcome measurement criteria

☐ Voiding at least every 4 hours while awake

☐ Urine output of more than 150 ml each time the patient
voids

☐ Absence of palpable bladder distention

☐ Urine output that approximates fluid intake

☐ Use of proper hygiene measures to decrease urinary
tract contamination

☐ Use of techniques to promote voiding

☐ Verbalization of understanding of postpartal diuresis

☐ Less than 50 ml of residual urine

☐ Absence of an abnormal level of bacteria in the urine

Key interventions

- Assess the patient's risk of uterine distention by noting the time of delivery in relation to her last voiding, I.V. and oral fluid intake, delivery method, type of anesthesia, and infant's size.

- Apply ice, as ordered, to the perineum immediately after delivery to decrease edema that may interfere with voiding.

- Palpate for bladder distention at least every 4 hours until the patient establishes an effective voiding pattern.

- Encourage the patient to void spontaneously in the first 6 to 8 hours after delivery. Measure urine output for the first 24 postpartal hours.

- Remind the patient to try to void every 2 to 4 hours while awake after the initial postpartal voiding. Encourage her not to delay voiding when she feels the urge.

- Promote voiding by helping the patient to the bathroom or bedside commode or placing her on a bedpan if she cannot ambulate.

- Stimulate voiding by running water in the sink, pouring warm water over the patient's perineum, or helping her to sit in a sitz bath to void.

- Teach the patient to rock slowly back and forth on the commode to promote complete bladder emptying.

- Monitor and document fluid intake and output. Teach the patient and her family how to help document intake and output.

- Teach the patient that proper handwashing and perineal hygiene can decrease the risk of urinary tract infection.

- Advise the patient to use a cleansing solution, such as diluted povidone-iodine (Betadine) solution or mild soap solution, on the perineum after each voiding to decrease bacterial contamination. Teach her how to rinse and dry her perineum gently after cleaning.

- Inform the patient about the normal postpartal fluid shift that causes diuresis. Explain that increased urination is not a sign of complications but of postpartal adaptation.

- Catheterize the patient who may have incomplete bladder emptying, as ordered, using an in-and-out technique to check for residual urine. If residual urine exceeds 50 ml, notify the health care professional.

- Insert a straight catheter for the patient who cannot void, as ordered. Document the amount of urine attained on catheterization. If this amount meets or exceeds 900 ml, clamp the catheter and then unclamp it in 1 hour. Notify the health care professional of findings.

- Obtain urine specimens for urinalysis and culture and sensitivity testing as ordered.

Venous thrombosis

Presence of a thrombus in a superficial or deep vein, which may cause inflammation of the vein wall (thrombophlebitis) or may cause no inflammation (phlebothrombosis).

NURSING DIAGNOSIS

Altered peripheral tissue perfusion related to obstruction of venous circulation secondary to venous thrombosis

DESIRED PATIENT OUTCOME

The patient will display improved peripheral tissue perfusion

Outcome measurement criteria

- ☐ Verbalization of the risks associated with venous thrombosis
- ☐ Adherence to activity limitations
- ☐ Demonstration of safe positioning
- ☐ Avoidance of massage of the affected area
- ☐ Use of heat therapy to the affected area
- ☐ Use of thigh-high supportive stockings
- ☐ Peripheral pulses of 2+ bilaterally
- ☐ Warm legs
- ☐ Rapid capillary refill time
- ☐ Absence of pallor of the affected leg
- ☐ Absence of signs and symptoms of pulmonary embolus

Key interventions

- Assess the patient's knowledge about venous thrombosis. Explain the risk of pulmonary embolus development.

- Discuss the importance of bed rest in decreasing the risk of pulmonary embolus, which can occur if a clot is dislodged.

- Promote bed rest by placing the bedside table, telephone, and call bell within easy reach; placing the infant's crib close to the side of the bed; and providing reading or activity materials as desired. Check the patient frequently to assess her needs.

- Explain the effects of positioning on venous circulation. Elevate the affected leg on pillows to decrease edema and prevent venous stasis.

- Teach the patient not to use the knee-gatch on the bed and not to cross her legs; both of these positions inhibit venous return.

- Encourage the patient to turn in bed frequently to decrease the risk of venous stasis in other body areas and to decrease discomfort caused by immobility.

- Caution the patient not to massage the affected area. Massage may loosen part of the clot and cause a pulmonary embolus.

- Apply warm, moist heat to the affected area as ordered to promote circulation. Check for proper functioning of a mechanical heating device at least every 8 hours. Assess the patient's skin temperature under the heating device at least every 4 hours.

- Apply thigh-high supportive elastic stockings as ordered. Explain that these stockings promote venous return and must remain in place throughout the course of treatment.

- Check and document the patient's peripheral pulses at least every 4 hours. Be alert for pulse weakening in the affected limb.

- Assess and document the temperature, color, and capillary refill time of bilateral extremities every 4 hours. Notify the health care professional of signs of increasing venous obstruction, such as increased coolness or pallor or decreased capillary refill time.

- Administer an antibiotic as prescribed for venous inflammation caused by infection. Teach the patient about its dosage schedule, benefits, and adverse effects.

- Assess the patient for signs and symptoms of pulmonary embolus: sudden onset of dyspnea, apprehension, tachypnea, chest pain, diaphoresis, pallor, tachycardia, hypotension, coughing, hemoptysis, pleural friction rub, and crackles.

- Notify the health care professional immediately of signs and symptoms of pulmonary embolus.

NURSING DIAGNOSIS

High risk for injury related to abnormal bleeding secondary to anticoagulant therapy

DESIRED PATIENT OUTCOME

The patient will remain free from injury resulting from abnormal bleeding

Outcome measurement criteria

☐ Verbalization of the need for anticoagulant therapy

☐ Prothrombin time (PT) and partial thromboplastin time (PTT) within therapeutic ranges

☐ Absence of signs of bleeding, such as hematuria, blood in stools, epistaxis, severe ecchymosis, bleeding from oral mucous membranes, and increased lochia flow

☐ Identification of signs and symptoms to report to the health care professional

☐ Description of ways to decrease the risk of abnormal bleeding

Key interventions

- Teach the patient about the need for and effects of anticoagulants. Teach her that anticoagulants do not dissolve clots but decrease the likelihood of further clot formation.

- Notify the patient that anticoagulant therapy probably will continue for several weeks after discharge.

- Review PT and PTT reports. With heparin (Liquaemin), the patient's PTT should be 2.5 to 3 times the control; with warfarin (Coumadin), PT should be 1.5 to 2 times the control. Teach the patient the significance of these values.

- Teach the patient about the adverse effects of anticoagulant therapy, and describe signs and symptoms to report to the health care professional.

- Assess urine color. Teach the patient to report urine that appears pink or orange.

- Obtain a urine specimen for urinalysis as ordered. Report the presence of red blood cells in the specimen.

- Teach the patient to evaluate her stool color and to report black, red, or pink stools immediately because they may signal occult or overt GI bleeding.

- Test stools for blood as ordered.

- Evaluate the patient's history for nosebleeds. Teach her to avoid disrupting the integrity of her nasal mucous membranes and to report epistaxis.

- Inspect the patient for ecchymosis, noting the size of ecchymotic areas and comparing them to previous assessments. Notify the health care professional of increasing ecchymosis.

- Teach the patient to monitor ecchymosis at home every day. During anticoagulant therapy, encourage her to avoid behaviors that can increase bruising, such as sports and careless movements.

- Observe the patient's oral mucous membranes every 8 hours and after mouth care during hospitalization. Instruct her to use only a soft-bristled toothbrush during anticoagulant therapy.

- Explain the risk of bleeding from oral mucous membranes, and teach the patient how to assess herself for such bleeding. Encourage her to avoid brittle foods that may disrupt the integrity of the oral mucous membranes.

- Evaluate the color, amount, and consistency of lochia. Notify the health care professional of increased bleeding.

- Teach the patient to recognize normal postpartal lochia and to report increased lochia flow or abnormal lochia flow.

- Evaluate venipuncture and injection sites for abnormal bleeding. Apply firm pressure to the sites for 5 to 10 minutes after venipuncture or injection. Report bleeding that lasts more than 10 minutes.

- Instruct the patient to avoid interrupting skin integrity. Teach her to cut her fingernails short, avoid scratching her skin, and use an electric razor when shaving.

- Caution the patient to avoid over-the-counter (OTC) drugs that contain aspirin or nonsteroidal anti-inflammatory drugs, which may increase bleeding time. Recommend that she check with the health care professional before using any OTC drug.

- Encourage the patient to obtain and wear a medical identification bracelet during anticoagulant therapy.

- Emphasize the need for the patient to attend all follow-up visits for evaluation of anticoagulant therapy.

- Stress the importance of notifying the health care professional if bleeding occurs and lasts more than 10 minutes.

- Teach self-administration of subcutaneous heparin injections if heparin is prescribed. Reassure the breast-feeding patient that heparin is safe to take when breast-feeding.

- Arrange for home visits as ordered for the patient on anticoagulant therapy.

NURSING DIAGNOSIS

Pain related to the effects of venous thrombosis

DESIRED PATIENT OUTCOME

The patient will report decreased pain

Outcome measurement criteria

☐ Use of pharmacologic and nonpharmacologic pain-relief measures

☐ Absence of signs and symptoms of pain

☐ Report of feeling adequately rested

☐ Report of decreased or absent pain

Key interventions

- Help the patient communicate her pain perception accurately. Ask her to rate her pain on a scale of 1 to 10 with 10 being the worst and 1 being the least.

- Observe for nonverbal signs of pain, such as grimacing, limited movement, guarding, and rapid or shallow breathing.

- Administer analgesics as prescribed.

- Teach the patient about the administration schedule, benefits, and adverse effects of prescribed analgesics.

- Teach the breast-feeding patient about the safety of breast-feeding during analgesic therapy. If breast-feeding must be interrupted, teach her how to use a breast pump to continue milk production through the acute phase of illness.

- Explain that pain is easier to relieve if it does not become severe before intervention. Encourage the patient to request analgesics frequently enough to control the pain.

- Teach the patient about nonpharmacologic pain-relief methods, such as relaxation and deep-breathing exercises and heat application.

- Offer back rubs to promote relaxation. Change bed linens as frequently as needed to maintain a clean, dry bed.

- Help the patient reposition herself in the bed every 2 to 4 hours. Provide pillows for support and for propping up the affected leg.

- Describe the importance of adequate rest in promoting healing. Limit visitors and decrease environmental stimuli to promote rest.

- Reassure the patient that the pain is temporary and will resolve as venous thrombosis abates.

- Reassess periodically to check for consistency between signs and reports of pain and those of rest and comfort.

Caput succedaneum

Fetal scalp edema caused by pressure during labor.

NURSING DIAGNOSIS

Anxiety (parental) related to lack of knowledge about caput succedaneum

DESIRED PATIENT OUTCOME

The parents will display comfort with the infant's appearance and demonstrate knowledge about caput succedaneum

Outcome measurement criteria

☐ Verbalization of an understanding of the disorder's cause

☐ Verbalization of an understanding of the disorder's management and prognosis

☐ Demonstration of attachment behaviors

Key interventions

• Teach the parents that caput succedaneum commonly results from fetal scalp pressure during labor and delivery. Explain how increased pressure can occur, such as by prolonged engagement of the fetus's head or use of a vacuum extractor.

• Reassure the parents that the disorder is benign and that it usually subsides without intervention during the first week after birth. Explain that the infant's head will become more symmetrical every day.

- Encourage the parents not to be afraid to touch the infant's head because of caput succedaneum. Demonstrate appropriate nurturing behaviors, as needed.

- Encourage the parents to discuss their feelings about the infant's appearance.

- Observe for persistent signs of lack of attachment, such as emotional withdrawal from the infant, resistance to infant care, distortion of the prognosis, or fear of taking the infant home.

- Refer the family with attachment difficulties to community agencies as needed.

Cardiovascular defect, congenital

Any structural defect of the heart, great vessels, or both that exists at birth. Defects may include atrial septal defect, aortic stenosis, coarctation of the aorta, complete transposition of the great vessels, hypoplastic left heart, patent ductus arteriosus, tetralogy of Fallot, and ventricular septal defect.

NURSING DIAGNOSIS

High risk for injury related to the physiologic effects of a congenital cardiovascular defect

DESIRED PATIENT OUTCOME

The infant will remain free from injury caused by a cardiovascular defect

Outcome measurement criteria

☐ Absence of signs and symptoms of infection

☐ Adequate oxygenation as evidenced by appropriate skin color

☐ Absence of respiratory distress

☐ Adequate weight gain

Key interventions

• Be alert for factors that increase the infant's risk of having cardiovascular defects, such as a family history of such defects; advanced maternal age; maternal exposure to drugs, alcohol, or infections such as rubella; and presence of other congenital anomalies.

• Perform a thorough initial assessment to establish a baseline and perform ongoing assessments to detect changes.

- Observe and document the infant's activity level. Note limb flaccidity, poor muscle tone, or lack of flexed positioning.

- Assess the infant's color, noting persistent acrocyanosis, cyanosis, pallor, mottling, or grayness. Watch for color changes with increased activity.

- Observe for general diaphoresis or localized sweating on the upper lip or across the brow.

- Assess the infant's respiratory effort. Check for signs of respiratory distress, such as dyspnea when supine, nasal flaring, grunting, or sternal retractions.

- Count respirations for a full minute while the infant is at rest. Document tachypnea (more than 60 breaths/minute).

- Auscultate the lungs to detect adventitious breath sounds.

- Assess for coolness in the arms and legs and check the presence and strength of the peripheral pulses.

- Count the apical pulse for 1 minute, particularly noting tachycardia (more than 160 beats/minute) or irregular rhythm.

- Auscultate for heart murmurs and bruits. Palpate for thrills around the heart.

- Assess blood pressure in all arms and legs. Marked differences may indicate coarctation of the aorta.

- Assess the infant's tolerance of feedings. Determine if feeding causes respiratory distress, color changes, onset of diaphoresis, or decreased muscle tone.

- Notify the health care professional immediately if signs of injury result from the congenital cardiovascular defect.

- Continue to assess and support the infant until a plan for management is developed and initiated.

NURSING DIAGNOSIS

Altered cardiopulmonary tissue perfusion related to decreased circulating oxygen secondary to a congenital cardiovascular defect

DESIRED PATIENT OUTCOME

The infant will display signs of adequate circulating oxygen

Outcome measurement criteria

☐ Respiratory rate of 30 to 60 breaths/minute

☐ Heart rate of 100 to 160 beats/minute

☐ Normal cardiac rhythm

☐ Blood pressure above 60/40 mm Hg peripherally or a mean of 30 mm Hg with umbilical artery catheter monitoring

☐ Pulse oximetry value of 95% or higher

☐ Capillary refill time of less than 4 seconds

☐ Absence of increasing cyanosis

☐ Age-appropriate arterial blood gas (ABG) levels

☐ Blood pH level of 7.31 to 7.45

☐ Urine output of at least 20 ml per day

Key interventions

• Monitor the infant's respiratory rate and effort. Report signs of increasing respiratory distress, such as sternal retractions, grunting, and nasal flaring.

• Administer oxygen as prescribed, using an oxygen hood, nasal continuous positive airway pressure, or endotracheal tube.

• Electronically monitor the infant's heart rate and rhythm. Document findings and report increasing tachycardia or the onset of bradycardia.

- Document pulse oximetry values. Observe for decreasing oxygen saturation levels.

- Monitor ABG levels as prescribed and report increasing acidosis, hypercapnia, or hypoxia.

- Monitor the infant's skin color and report increasing cyanosis.

- Assess and document capillary refill time. Observe for increasing capillary refill time—a sign of decreasing oxygenation.

- Assess urine output, weighing diapers or bedding to obtain an estimate. Document fluid intake and urine output.

- Administer I.V. fluids as prescribed, using a volume-control delivery system.

- Administer a vasopressor, diuretic, or digoxin as prescribed to maintain adequate circulating oxygen.

NURSING DIAGNOSIS

High risk for altered nutrition: less than body requirements, related to fatigue and dyspnea during feedings

DESIRED PATIENT OUTCOME

The infant will obtain sufficient nutrients to support growth

Outcome measurement criteria

☐ Weight gain of 0.4 to 0.5 oz (10 to 15 g) per day in a preterm infant; 0.7 to 1.1 oz (20 to 30 g) per day in a full-term infant

☐ Intake of 110 to 150 calories/kg/day

Key interventions

- Weigh the infant at the same time every day, using the same scale. Document weight changes so that the infant's progress can be tracked easily.

- Offer frequent, small feedings using a soft nipple with a large hole. Provide frequent rest periods during feedings for the infant who develops slight dyspnea, cyanosis, or diaphoresis.

- Begin gavage feedings as ordered if the infant cannot consume about 1 oz (30 ml) of formula within 30 minutes or if the infant develops tachypnea during oral feedings.

- Increase the formula's caloric content as prescribed to decrease the risk of fluid overload while meeting caloric needs.

- Document the infant's response to each feeding.

NURSING DIAGNOSIS

Activity intolerance related to inadequate circulating oxygen

DESIRED PATIENT OUTCOME

The infant will display increasing tolerance of feedings and other activities

Outcome measurement criteria

☐ Appearance of restfulness during quiet periods

☐ Infrequent periods of crying

☐ Absence of pallor or cyanosis during activity

☐ Decreased dyspnea with feedings

Key interventions

• Provide a thermally neutral, oxygen-rich environment for the infant to reduce physiologic stress.

• Cluster nursing activities to provide long, frequent rest periods for the infant.

• Observe to determine if the infant sleeps restfully or is restless. If the infant is restless, monitor the environment and reduce external and internal stressors, such as cold room temperature, hunger, or physical discomfort.

• Administer a cardiac glycoside as prescribed to increase cardiac output.

• Anticipate the infant's needs to help prevent crying, which may lead to fatigue and dyspnea.

• Gradually increase the infant's activity. Observe for changes in color and vital signs during activity.

• Use small, frequent feedings with a soft, large-hole nipple to assist with energy conservation.

• Document the infant's response to activity.

NURSING DIAGNOSIS

Ineffective family coping: compromised, related to grief over the loss of the idealized infant and guilt, fear, anxiety, and lack of knowledge about the infant's condition

DESIRED PATIENT OUTCOME

The family will cope effectively with and adapt positively to their loss and their infant's special needs

Outcome measurement criteria

☐ Demonstration of progress through stages of grief

☐ Absence of assigned guilt or blame among family members

☐ Demonstration of emotional support among family members

☐ Verbalization of an accurate understanding of the infant's condition

☐ Verbalization of an understanding of the infant's prognosis and treatment plan

☐ Involvement in the infant's care

☐ Demonstration of safe care of the infant

☐ Demonstration of attachment behaviors

Key interventions

• Establish a supportive, caring environment when the family initially is informed of the infant's condition. Allow time for family members to express initial concerns. Encourage them to ask questions; answer briefly and factually in the initial stages.

• Facilitate early family visits with the infant.

• Help the family explore the infant. Point out positive aspects of the infant's body and well-being.

• Teach the family about the infant's need for increased rest.

• Briefly and simply explain the monitoring and oxygen equipment.

• When feasible, touch the infant gently and lovingly to demonstrate acceptance of the infant for family members who may be experiencing shock, fear, and withdrawal. Teach them how to touch the infant, if necessary.

• Encourage the family to tape their soothing voices for the infant. Explain that the tape will be played during the infant's daily care.

• Provide an accepting environment for the family to express their feelings and fears. Help them recognize that part of their response is normal grief. Assist them in feeling comfortable with their shock, anger, disbelief, denial, depression, or withdrawal.

- Encourage family members to share their feelings and concerns with each other and health care team members frequently. Remind them not to become victims of persistent feelings of guilt or blame.

- Encourage family members to be supportive of each other. Reinforce that each individual's adaptation is unique.

- When the family is ready for further knowledge about their infant's treatment and prognosis, help them obtain accurate information.

- Arrange a visit with the family of another child with a congenital cardiovascular defect, if the family desires.

- Encourage family members to take an active role in the infant's care. Facilitate visits whenever they desire.

- Teach family members how to feed the infant safely. Demonstrate the use of appropriate feeding techniques and equipment. Teach other infant care skills, such as diapering, bathing, and providing cord care.

- Explain the need for family members to learn infant cardiopulmonary resuscitation. Provide information about class schedules and locations and encourage them to participate.

- Observe for persistent signs of lack of attachment, such as emotional withdrawal from the infant, resistance to infant care, distortion of the prognosis, or fear of taking the infant home.

- Refer the family with attachment difficulties to community agencies as needed.

- Encourage the family to become involved with a support group for parents of infants with congenital cardiovascular defects.

Cephalhematoma

Collection of blood between the skull bone and periosteum, accompanied by swelling of the affected cranial bone.

NURSING DIAGNOSIS

Anxiety (parental) related to lack of knowledge about cephalhematoma

DESIRED PATIENT OUTCOME

The parents will display reduced anxiety about the infant and increased knowledge about cephalhematoma

Outcome measurement criteria

☐ Verbalization of an understanding of cephalhematoma's cause, management, and prognosis

☐ Identification of the risks associated with cephalhematoma

☐ Demonstration of techniques used to assess for jaundice

☐ Demonstration of attachment behaviors

Key interventions

- Teach the parents that cephalhematoma is caused by excessive pressure on the head during labor and delivery. Explain that rupture of a small blood vessel causes blood to collect, forming the characteristic bulge.

- Inform the parents that cephalhematomas usually are largest on the 2nd or 3rd day after birth and typically resolve without treatment in 2 weeks to 3 months.

- Advise the parents that cephalhematoma does not indicate brain damage, but that it somewhat increases the infant's risk of hyperbilirubinemia because of the breakdown of red blood cells collected between the skull and periosteum.

- Demonstrate how to assess the infant's skin, sclera, and mucous membranes for a golden or yellow appearance. Teach the parents how to blanch the skin with finger pressure and observe for a yellow appearance before normal skin color returns. Instruct them to do this daily at home, using adequate natural light.

- Encourage the parents not to be afraid to touch the infant's head because of cephalhematoma.

- Observe for persistent signs of lack of attachment, such as emotional withdrawal from the infant, resistance to infant care, distortion of the prognosis, or fear of taking the infant home.

- Refer the family with attachment difficulties to community agencies as needed.

- Teach the parents to promote bilirubin breakdown by occasionally exposing the infant to natural sunlight. Reinforce the need to keep the infant warm during such exposure.

Circumcision

Surgical excision of the prepuce of the penis.

NURSING DIAGNOSIS
High risk for injury related to the effects of circumcision

DESIRED PATIENT OUTCOME
The infant will remain free from circumcision-induced injury

Outcome measurement criteria
☐ Absence of excessive penile bleeding

☐ Absence of penile adhesion to diapers or dressings

☐ Urine output within normal limits

☐ Absence of signs of penile infection

Key interventions
- Check the penis for bleeding hourly for the first 12 hours after circumcision. Spots of blood are common during the first few hours, but all bleeding should subside within a few hours. If bleeding occurs, apply gentle intermittent pressure to the penis with a sterile gauze pad and notify the health care professional.

- Immediately after circumcision, apply a generous amount of prescribed ointment to a sterile gauze pad or use a sterile wrap permeated with a petroleum substance and wrap the penis. Diaper the infant loosely.

- Reapply ointment every 4 hours or with each diaper change until healing occurs so that the penis does not stick to the diaper or dressing. To avoid obstruction of the urethral meatus, apply ointment in a thin layer on the tip of the penis.

- For circumcisions performed with a bell-shaped plastic device (Plastibell), do not apply a dressing; simply diaper the infant loosely.

- Check the infant's urine output and color and adequacy of the urine stream. Edema and trauma to the glans may cause difficult or painful voiding. Notify the health care professional if the infant has not voided within 4 hours of circumcision.

- As the circumcision heals, observe for signs of infection, such as localized redness and edema, inability to void, purulent discharge, fever, lethargy, tachypnea, and tachycardia. Notify the health care professional if infection is suspected.

NURSING DIAGNOSIS

Anxiety (parental) related to lack of knowledge about appropriate care for the newly circumcised infant

DESIRED PATIENT OUTCOME

The parents will display reduce anxiety and increased knowledge about care of the infant's penis

Outcome measurement criteria

☐ Verbalization of appropriate methods of caring for the circumcised penis

☐ Demonstration of safe techniques for care

☐ Identification of signs of normal healing and of danger

Key interventions

- Teach the parents that the infant may be irritable and may eat poorly for the first few hours after circumcision. Encourage them to provide soothing care for the infant.

- Help the parents inspect the newly circumcised penis. Explain that the dark red appearance of the glans is normal after circumcision and will diminish as healing occurs.

- If a bell-shaped plastic device (Plastibell) was used, explain that the device maintains gentle pressure on the glans and will remain in place until healing is complete.

- Caution the parents not to try to dislodge the bell-shaped plastic device (Plastibell). Advise them that it should fall off in about 1 week; if it remains in place after 8 days, they should contact the health care professional.

- If the glans is exposed, explain the importance of keeping the area around the penis clean to decrease the risk of infection, for example, by changing the infant's diaper at least every 4 hours.

- Teach the parents to clean the penis without creating undue friction on the glans. Instruct them to clean the area by squeezing warm water over the glans at each diaper change. When more vigorous cleaning is needed to remove feces from the penis, teach them to gently wipe the soiled area with a soft cloth saturated with water only. Advise them to avoid commercially prepared wipes because they may contain alcohol.

- Teach the parents to apply a loose dressing to the end of the penis at each diaper change. The dressing may be a gauze permeated with petroleum ointment, a sterile gauze pad that has had ointment applied, or a loose gauze dressing, which is used when ointment is applied directly to the glans.

- Encourage the parents to use sufficient ointment to prevent the penis from sticking to the diaper or gauze pad, but not so much ointment that it blocks the urethral meatus.

- If the infant's penis becomes stuck, teach the parents to squeeze water over the area until the diaper or gauze pad can be loosened without damaging the penis.

- Explain the importance of keeping the infant's diapers loose for the first 3 to 4 days after circumcision to promote comfort.

- Inform the parents that granulation normally occurs during healing and that the glans normally develops a yellowish exudate within 24 hours. Advise them not to dislodge the exudate or worry that it is a sign of infection.

- Instruct the parents to note their infant's voiding pattern and to contact the health care professional if the infant cannot void.

- Teach the parents to notify the health care professional if the circumcision site starts to bleed, if the penis develops edema and erythema, or if the infant develops a fever, becomes lethargic, or refuses feedings.

Cleft lip or palate

Congenital interruption of the upper lip, upper palate, or both.

NURSING DIAGNOSIS

High risk for altered nutrition: less than body requirements, related to inability to suck adequately

DESIRED PATIENT OUTCOME

The infant will obtain sufficient nutrition to allow normal growth and development

Outcome measurement criteria

☐ Caloric intake of about 110 to 120 calories/kg/day

☐ Fluid intake of about 140 to 160 ml/kg/day

☐ Weight gain of about 1 oz (28 g)/day in the first 6 months after the initial recovery of birth weight

☐ Absence of vomiting and fatigue after feeding

Key interventions

- Document whether the infant has a complete or partial cleft lip, palate, or both after the initial assessment.

- For the infant with a partial cleft palate, assess the ability to suck by gently placing a clean, gloved finger in the mouth and directing the finger pad toward the palate.

- Calculate the infant's caloric and fluid needs; document calculations for daily recommended intake.

- Maintain daily records of food and fluid intake and urine and stool output.

- Hold the infant in an upright or sitting position during feedings to decrease the risk of aspiration.

- For a breast-fed infant, teach the mother to soften the areola by rubbing it with expressed milk, to hold the nipple to the side of the infant's mouth during feedings, and to use a breast shield designed for use by an infant with cleft lip or palate, if needed. Assess the infant for adequate sucking during breast-feeding. If the infant cannot create sufficient suction, recommend that the mother pump her breast milk for the infant.

- For a bottle-fed infant, teach the parents to use a nipple that is specially designed for premature infants; place the nipple at the side and back of the infant's mouth; and avoid removing the nipple from the mouth unnecessarily during feedings.

- Teach the parents to provide small, slow, frequent feedings; longer feedings may exhaust the infant. Advise them to burp the infant frequently, because large amounts of air are ingested while swallowing.

- Instruct the parents to give the infant water at the end of each feeding to rinse the oral cavity slightly.

- Teach the parents to gently clean the infant's face after feeding to avoid contaminating nasal mucous membranes.

- Weigh the infant daily and document findings.

- Adjust daily intake calculations as needed based on the infant's weight gain.

NURSING DIAGNOSIS

High risk for aspiration related to an inability to clear secretions or milk from the cleft palate and nasal mucous membranes

DESIRED PATIENT OUTCOME
The infant will not aspirate secretions or feedings

Outcome measurement criteria
- ☐ Respiratory rate of 30 to 60 breaths/minute
- ☐ Absence of signs of respiratory distress
- ☐ Absence of dyspnea and cyanosis
- ☐ Normal breath sounds on auscultation
- ☐ Pulse oximetry values of 95% or more
- ☐ Absence of signs of respiratory infection
- ☐ Absence of excessive nasopharyngeal secretions

Key interventions
- Assess the infant's respiratory status, counting respirations for 1 minute. Document findings.
- Observe for and document signs of respiratory distress, such as nasal flaring, grunting, shallow respirations, and sternal retractions.
- Observe for and document dyspnea or cyanosis.
- Record pulse oximetry values.
- Clear the infant's oropharynx and nasopharynx with gentle suctioning, as needed.
- Position the infant on the side in the crib with the head elevated 30 degrees to decrease the risk of secretion accumulation in the pharynx.
- Auscultate the lungs and document any adventitious breath sounds.
- Notify the health care professional of adventitious breath sounds or persistent signs of respiratory distress.
- Keep suction and resuscitation equipment nearby during feedings.

NURSING DIAGNOSIS

Ineffective family coping: compromised, related to grief over the loss of the idealized infant and guilt, fear, anxiety, and lack of knowledge about the infant's condition

DESIRED PATIENT OUTCOME

The family will cope effectively with and adapt positively to their loss and their infant's special needs

Outcome measurement criteria

- ☐ Demonstration of progress through stages of grief
- ☐ Absence of assigned guilt or blame among family members
- ☐ Demonstration of emotional support among family members
- ☐ Verbalization of an accurate understanding of the infant's condition
- ☐ Verbalization of an understanding of the infant's prognosis and treatment plan
- ☐ Involvement in the infant's care
- ☐ Demonstration of safe care of the infant
- ☐ Demonstration of attachment behaviors

Key interventions

- Establish a supportive relationship with family members. Encourage them to ask questions; answer briefly and factually in the initial stages.
- Facilitate early family interaction with the infant after they have been told of the infant's cleft lip or palate.
- Help the family explore the infant. Point out positive aspects of the infant's body and well-being. Reinforce that surgical correction for cleft lip and palate is highly successful.

- Handle the infant gently and lovingly to demonstrate acceptance of the infant for family members who may be experiencing shock, fear, and withdrawal.

- Provide an accepting environment for the family to express their feelings and fears. Help them recognize that part of their response is normal grief. Assist them in feeling comfortable with their shock, anger, disbelief, denial, depression, or withdrawal.

- Encourage family members to share their feelings and concerns with each other and health care team members frequently. Remind them not to become victims of persistent feelings of guilt or blame.

- Encourage family members to be compassionate and supportive with each other. Reinforce that each individual's adaptation is unique.

- When the family is ready for further knowledge about their infant's treatment and prognosis, help them obtain accurate information. Use pictures to help them visualize the effects of complete repair. Answer their questions and provide written information as needed.

- Arrange a visit with the family of another child with cleft lip and palate, if the family desires.

- Encourage family members to take an active role in the infant's care as much as possible. Facilitate visits whenever they desire.

- Teach family members how to feed the infant safely. Demonstrate the use of appropriate feeding techniques and equipment.

- Show family members how to gently suction the infant's oropharynx and nasopharynx to prevent aspiration.

- Teach other infant care skills, such as diapering, bathing, and providing cord care.

- Observe for persistent signs of lack of attachment, such as emotional withdrawal from the infant, resistance to infant care, distortion of the prognosis, or fear of taking the infant home.

- Refer the family with attachment difficulties to social services or other community agencies as needed. Promote the use of these supports.

- Encourage the family to become involved with a support group for parents of infants with congenital defects.

Cold stress

Excessive heat loss that causes the body to use compensatory mechanisms to maintain the core temperature.

NURSING DIAGNOSIS

Ineffective thermoregulation related to the infant's immature thermoregulatory mechanisms

DESIRED PATIENT OUTCOME

The infant will maintain a core temperature of 97.7° to 99.5° F (36.5° to 37.5° C)

Outcome measurement criteria

☐ Presence of a thermally neutral environment

☐ Absence of tachypnea

☐ Absence of deepening acrocyanosis or cyanosis

Key interventions

• Assess the infant's temperature at birth and once every hour until stable. In the nonstressed full-term infant, the body temperature should become stable within 12 hours after birth.

• Immediately after birth, place the infant in a prewarmed radiant warmer or incubator to decrease heat loss by conduction.

• Dry the infant well after birth and maintain dry skin to decrease heat loss by evaporation.

• Remove damp blankets or towels from contact with the infant.

- For the high-risk or preterm infant, cover the radiant warmer with plastic wrap to maintain a draft-free environment.

- Place the stable, dry infant in skin-to-skin contact with the mother to help maintain the infant's body temperature.

- Observe and document the infant's respiratory rate, particularly noting tachypnea, which results from increased oxygen demands as a result of cold stress.

- Observe for increasing acrocyanosis or generalized cyanosis, which may signal an inability to meet increased oxygen demands.

- Assess the infant's oral mucous membranes for color changes to evaluate cyanosis or acrocyanosis more thoroughly.

- Keep the nursery's ambient temperature at about 75° F (23.8° C).

- Keep the stabilized infant clothed and wrapped as needed to help maintain an appropriate core body temperature and decrease heat loss by convection.

- Use the axillary method for routine assessment of the stabilized infant's temperature.

- Explain to the parents that temperature maintenance is critical to the infant's survival; teach them how to take an axillary temperature.

- Teach the parents that skin temperature changes can easily alter the infant's core temperature. Encourage them to cover the infant's skin well when exposure to a cool environment is likely. Explain that the infant has an immature shivering mechanism for thermogenesis and that a healthy infant who is cold commonly cries and becomes very active to generate heat.

Nursing Diagnosis

High risk for injury related to hyperthermia secondary to correction of hypothermia

DESIRED PATIENT OUTCOME

The infant will remain free from injury caused by correction of hypothermia

Outcome measurement criteria

☐ Absence of apnea

☐ Arterial blood gas (ABG) levels within normal limits

☐ Absence of skin temperature above 98° F (36.7° C)

Key interventions

- Warm the cold-stressed infant over 2 to 4 hours.

- Assess the infant's skin temperature by placing a thermistor probe on the abdomen between the umbilicus and pubis or on the skin over the liver. Do not place the probe over a bony prominence or on an arm or leg.

- Place the infant in an incubator and raise the incubator temperature gradually to warm the infant's skin temperature to about 98° F (36.7° C).

- Assess and document the infant's axillary temperature periodically.

- Monitor and document the infant's respiratory status, particularly noting decreased respiratory rate or apneic episodes.

- Report ABG levels as ordered; be alert for acidosis.

- Report apneic episodes or a skin temperature above 99.0° F (37.2° C).

- Wean the infant from the incubator over several hours or, for a high-risk or preterm infant, over several days.

- Dress the infant in an undershirt and diaper and gradually decrease the incubator temperature.

- Assess and document the temperature of the infant and the incubator. Assess the infant's respiratory and activity response to temperature changes.

- Decrease the incubator temperature gradually to match the nursery's ambient temperature. Cover the infant with blankets and open the incubator's portholes.

- Place the dressed and wrapped infant in an open crib when the core temperature has stabilized and the skin temperature is 97° to 98° F (36.1° to 36.7° C).

Gastrointestinal obstruction, congenital

Congenital anatomical disorder that causes abnormal functioning of the GI tract and commonly necessitates emergency surgery.

NURSING DIAGNOSIS

High risk for fluid volume deficit related to vomiting secondary to GI obstruction

DESIRED PATIENT OUTCOME

The infant will display adequate fluid volume

Outcome measurement criteria

☐ Appropriate skin turgor

☐ Absence of tachycardia

☐ Absence of projectile vomiting

☐ Urine specific gravity of 1.001 to 1.020

☐ Weight loss of no more than 10% of birth weight

☐ Stability of weight after initial recovery

☐ Serum electrolyte levels within normal limits

Key interventions

- Assess the infant's skin turgor, particularly noting skin tenting that previously was absent.

- Assess and document the infant's heart rate and pattern. Be alert for increasing tachycardia—a sign of hypovolemia.

- Monitor and document the infant's fluid intake and urine output. Weigh the infant's diapers to accurately estimate urine output. Estimate the volume of emesis.

- Observe the infant's bowel movements. Be alert for the absence of bowel movements after passage of the first stool.

- Note the force and color of emesis in the infant. Projectile vomiting of bile-colored or dark liquid indicates obstruction.

- Measure urine specific gravity as ordered.

- Weigh the infant daily and record findings. Observe for persistent weight loss.

- Notify the health care professional of signs of dehydration or abnormal fluid loss.

- Administer I.V. fluids as prescribed to support the infant's circulating fluid volume.

- Monitor laboratory test results as ordered and report abnormal findings. Be alert for alkalosis or hyperkalemia, which are complications of GI obstruction.

NURSING DIAGNOSIS

Impaired gas exchange related to GI distention that creates abnormal pressure in the lungs

DESIRED PATIENT OUTCOME

The infant will demonstrate effective respiratory gas exchange

Outcome measurement criteria

☐ Respiratory rate of 30 to 50 breaths/minute

☐ Absence of signs of respiratory distress

☐ Absence of cyanosis, ashen color, or increasing acrocyanosis

☐ Normal breath sounds on auscultation

☐ Age-appropriate arterial blood gas (ABG) levels

☐ Blood pH level of 7.31 to 7.45

☐ Pulse oximetry value of 95% or higher

Key interventions

- Assess and document the infant's respiratory rate and effort and signs of respiratory distress, such as nasal flaring, grunting, or sternal retractions.

- Observe the infant's color and monitor for changes.

- Auscultate the lungs for adventitious or absent breath sounds.

- Observe and measure the infant's abdominal girth, noting any abnormal increase. Auscultate for displaced bowel sounds.

- Auscultate the heart and assess for displacement of the point of maximal impulse.

- Assist with bowel decompression as ordered by inserting a nasogastric tube.

- Administer oxygen or assist with intubation as ordered.

- Assess the infant for signs of a diaphragmatic hernia. If breath sounds are absent on one side of the chest and abdominal girth is increased, avoid bag-and-mask ventilation because it may displace air into bowel segments herniated through the infant's diaphragm and increase respiratory distress.

- Monitor and report ABG and pulse oximetry values as ordered.

- Notify the health care professional of increasing abdominal girth, signs of respiratory distress, and deteriorating laboratory test results.

NURSING DIAGNOSIS

High risk for infection related to aspiration of vomitus

DESIRED PATIENT OUTCOME

The infant will show no signs or symptoms of aspiration pneumonia

Outcome measurement criteria

☐ Normal breath sounds on auscultation

☐ Axillary temperature below 98.6° F (37.0° C)

☐ Absence of tachycardia

☐ Absence of tachypnea or signs of respiratory distress

Key interventions

- Protect the infant from the risk of aspiration pneumonia. Use suction equipment as needed to maintain a patent airway, particularly after the infant vomits.

- Place the infant in a side-lying position to promote drainage of secretions from the oropharynx.

- Assess and document the infant's temperature and other vital signs. Monitor respiratory effort and breath sounds.

- Notify the health care professional of assessment findings that suggest infection.

- Administer antibiotics as prescribed.

NURSING DIAGNOSIS

Anxiety (parental) related to the unknown outcome of surgery

DESIRED PATIENT OUTCOME

The parents will cope effectively with their anxiety

Outcome measurement criteria

☐ Verbalization of fears and concerns about the infant's condition

☐ Expression of mutual support among family members

☐ Verbalization of an understanding of the treatment plan for GI obstruction

☐ Demonstration of attachment behaviors

Key interventions

• Establish a rapport with the infant's parents. Encourage them to discuss their feelings, ask questions, and identify concerns.

• Assess the parents' knowledge about GI obstruction in the infant. Offer as much information about its pathophysiology as they desire.

• Update the parents frequently about the infant's condition and progress.

• Help the parents obtain accurate information about their infant's prognosis.

• Demonstrate acceptance of the infant and teach the parents, as needed, about appropriate ways to touch and caress the infant.

• Teach the parents about any monitoring equipment being used.

• Observe for persistent signs of lack of attachment, such as emotional withdrawal from the infant, resistance to infant care, distortion of the prognosis, or fear of taking the infant home.

• Refer the family with attachment difficulties to community agencies as needed.

Hip dysplasia, congenital

Birth defect in which one or both hips have developed and function imperfectly.

NURSING DIAGNOSIS

Altered growth and development related to the effects of undiagnosed or untreated congenital hip dysplasia

DESIRED PATIENT OUTCOME

The infant will display age-appropriate growth and development and will receive appropriate treatment for congenital hip dysplasia

Outcome measurement criteria

☐ Maintenance of correct anatomical positioning of the hip

☐ Compliance with treatment for hip dysplasia

☐ Achievement of normal developmental milestones

Key interventions

- Assess for factors associated with a high risk of congenital hip dysplasia, such as breech presentation, presence of other congenital anomalies, and a family history of congenital hip dysplasia.

- Assess the infant for signs of hip dysplasia, such as asymmetrical gluteal and thigh folds, legs, knees, or leg movements.

- Document abnormal findings and notify the health care professional.

- Help the health care professional perform Barlow's maneuver as needed and listen for Ortolani's sign (clicking when the head of the femur moves in or out of the acetabulum).

- Place triple diapers on the infant with congenital hip dysplasia as ordered, to maintain proper hip abduction.

- Assist with application of a Pavlik harness as ordered.

- Assist with care of the infant in a hip spica cast if used.

- Provide appropriate verbal, visual, tactile, and auditory stimulation for the infant in an abduction device.

NURSING DIAGNOSIS

Ineffective family coping: compromised, related to grief over the loss of the idealized child and to the need for an abduction device

DESIRED PATIENT OUTCOME

The family will cope effectively with feelings about the infant's condition and will effectively manage the infant's care

Outcome measurement criteria

- ☐ Verbalization of feelings about the infant's condition
- ☐ Demonstration of mutual support among family members
- ☐ Description of the anatomy associated with congenital hip dysplasia
- ☐ Demonstration of appropriate care of the infant in an abduction device
- ☐ Demonstration of appropriate social stimulation of the infant
- ☐ Demonstration of adequate nurturing behavior

Key interventions

- Establish a supportive relationship with the family. Encourage them to express their feelings about the infant's condition. Recognize their loss of the idealized infant and support them through grieving.

- Reassure the family that early treatment of congenital hip dysplasia typically is very successful, is relatively brief, and produces no adverse effects.

- Encourage family members to accept that everyone copes with grief and other feelings uniquely. Reinforce the need for mutual support.

- Encourage acceptance and promote attachment by emphasizing the infant's positive aspects.

- Discuss the anatomical condition and anticipated treatment associated with their infant's hip dysplasia. Provide written and verbal information when the family is ready.

- Emphasize the importance of maintaining abduction to ensure hip stability.

- Demonstrate how to apply triple diapers, as needed, putting them on snugly, but not too tightly.

- Demonstrate how to apply the Pavlik harness. Remind family members not to adjust the harness until the health care professional checks the infant. If the Pavlik harness is not to be removed, teach them how to sponge-bathe the infant.

- Teach family members to assess the skin under the harness daily for signs of irritation or breakdown. To reduce skin irritation, teach them to lightly pad harness areas that come in contact with bony prominences. Also instruct them to consult the health care professional before applying powders or lotions under the harness straps because these agents may further damage irritated skin.

- Allow extra time for teaching and reassuring the family whose infant will have a spica cast, because they may feel overwhelmed by this experience.

- After spica cast application, frequently monitor and document the infant's vital signs, skin color and temperature, peripheral pulses, capillary refill time in the toes and feet, and swelling in the legs. Report any abnormal findings. Reposition the infant at least every 2 hours while the cast dries. Leave the cast uncovered and use a cool fan to speed drying if the infant is sufficiently warm.

- Demonstrate appropriate feeding positions for the infant in a spica cast, such as the football-hold position for the breast-fed infant or the modified cradle-hold (with the cast on the family member's lap) or football-hold position for the bottle-fed infant.

- Teach the family to prevent skin contamination and irritation by the cast. Demonstrate how to petal the edges of the cast, using strips of tape, adhesive bandages, or strips of disposable diaper.

- Emphasize the need to keep the cast's perineal opening dry and clean. Demonstrate how to use a fluid barrier, such as plastic, at the perineal opening. Advise family members to tuck an infant-sized diaper smoothly into the edges of the cast at the opening and then place a much larger diaper over the entire diaper area of the cast.

- Help the family obtain a safely modified car seat to use while the infant has a cast.

- Teach the family about the infant's need for auditory, visual, and tactile stimulation. Encourage them to provide appropriate stimulation and to use safe methods of physical interaction with the infant.

- Provide information about support groups and counseling services. Encourage the family to use these services as needed.

Human immunodeficiency virus infection

Presence of the human immunodeficiency virus (HIV) in the infant's blood or tissues or presence of HIV antibodies, transmitted by the infected mother. The infant of an HIV-infected mother has a 25% to 30% chance of acquiring the virus, but the virus may not be evident for up to 2 years.

NURSING DIAGNOSIS

Altered protection related to the effects of the mother's HIV infection and the infant's immature immune system

DESIRED PATIENT OUTCOME

The infant will display no signs or symptoms of illness

Outcome measurement criteria

□ Vital signs within normal limits

□ Absence of signs of superficial infection

□ Absence of signs of sepsis

Key interventions

• Assess for factors that increase the infant's risk of HIV infection, such as maternal HIV infection, I.V. drug abuse, sexually transmitted disease, or inadequate pre-natal care. Keep in mind that an infant whose mother has the virus may test positive for HIV antibodies, but may not be infected.

• Strictly observe universal precautions.

• Prevent staff members and family members from caring for the infant if they are even mildly ill.

- Encourage the seropositive mother to avoid breast-feeding the infant because the virus can be transmitted through breast milk.

- Protect the infant from opportunistic infections by bathing the infant completely before administering vitamin K, providing meticulous care of the umbilical cord, and repositioning the infant frequently in the crib to prevent skin breakdown.

- Monitor the infant's vital signs and report signs of infection, such as tachypnea, tachycardia, apnea, and hypothermia.

- Observe for and initiate prompt treatment for signs of infection in the infant.

- Administer I.V. fluids and antibiotics as prescribed.

NURSING DIAGNOSIS

High risk for altered parenting related to the infant's potential illness and lack of information about effective parenting techniques

DESIRED PATIENT OUTCOME

The parents will care for the infant effectively and knowledgeably

Outcome measurement criteria

- ☐ Verbalization of an understanding of the infant's risk of developing HIV infection
- ☐ Demonstration of techniques for comforting the infant
- ☐ Verbalization of an understanding of the infant's need for rest
- ☐ Demonstration of effective techniques for infant feeding, bathing, and clothing
- ☐ Use of external resources to assist with infant care

Key interventions

- Establish a rapport with the infant's parents. Encourage them to discuss feelings, ask questions, and identify concerns.

- Explain that the infant has a 25% to 30% chance of acquiring HIV and that the virus may not be evident for up to 2 years.

- Teach the parents about different methods of comforting the infant to promote rest. Explain that, at times, the infant may be comforted by being caressed, rocked, cuddled, and talked to and that, at other times, the infant may be comforted by being swaddled and placed in an environment with little external stimuli. Explain how nonnutritive sucking can comfort the infant.

- Model nurturing behaviors, such as cuddling, swaddling, and caressing, and teach the parents how to perform them, as needed.

- Help the parents recognize signs of overstimulation, such as high-pitched crying, restlessness, and yawning. Encourage the parents to allow the infant frequent rest periods.

- Inform the parents of the infant's nutritional needs and feeding habits. Show them how to feed the infant appropriately.

- Teach the parents how to provide routine infant care, allowing the infant to rest between care activities. Encourage them to participate in the hospitalized infant's care and evaluate their interaction with the infant.

- Observe for persistent signs of lack of attachment, such as emotional withdrawal from the infant, resistance to infant care, distortion of the prognosis, or fear of taking the infant home.

- Encourage the infant's mother to discuss her plans for managing her seropositive status.

- Refer the parents to support services for parenting classes, home health agencies, and adoption or foster care services. Encourage them to use as many services as needed.

- Make referrals to child protective services and other social services as needed.

Hydrocephalus

Congenital condition characterized by cranial enlargement and caused by excessive accumulation of cerebrospinal fluid (CSF) in the ventricles of the brain.

NURSING DIAGNOSIS

High risk for injury related to increased head weight and size

DESIRED PATIENT OUTCOME

The infant will remain free from injury related to hydrocephalus

Outcome measurement criteria

☐ Full range of motion (ROM) in the arms and legs

☐ Absence of signs of tissue breakdown in areas of pressure on the head

☐ Absence of signs of local infection in areas of skin breakdown

Key interventions

• Provide extra support for the infant's head during procedures and interventions. Maintain proper positioning to ensure a patent airway when moving the infant.

• Use soft linens and an egg-crate mattress or sheepskin under the infant's head to decrease the risk of skin breakdown from pressure. Change the infant's head position every 2 hours to prevent breakdown.

• Perform passive ROM exercises on the arms and legs every 4 hours to decrease the risk of contracture.

- Promptly clean any vomitus after feeding, and ensure that skin creases are clean and dry.

- Observe for and document pink or reddened areas, which suggest the beginning of skin breakdown; position the infant to relieve pressure on these areas.

- Observe for and document increasing redness or drainage from a pressure site. Notify the health care professional of signs of increasing disruption of skin integrity.

NURSING DIAGNOSIS

Ineffective family coping: compromised, related to grief over the loss of the idealized infant and guilt, fear, anxiety, and lack of knowledge about hydrocephalus

DESIRED PATIENT OUTCOME

The family will cope effectively with their loss and will adapt positively to their infant's special needs

Outcome measurement criteria

☐ Demonstration of progress through stages of grief

☐ Absence of assigned guilt or blame among family members

☐ Demonstration of emotional support among family members

☐ Verbalization of an accurate understanding of the infant's condition

☐ Verbalization of an understanding of the infant's prognosis and treatment plan

☐ Involvement in the infant's care

☐ Demonstration of safe care of the infant

☐ Demonstration of attachment behaviors

Key interventions

- Establish a supportive, caring environment when the family initially is informed of the infant's condition. Allow time for family members to express initial concerns. Encourage them to ask questions; answer briefly and factually in the initial stages.

- Facilitate early family viewing and holding of the infant.

- Help the family explore the infant. Point out positive aspects of the infant's body and well-being.

- When feasible, touch the infant gently and lovingly to demonstrate acceptance of the infant for family members who may be experiencing shock, fear, and withdrawal. Teach them how to touch the infant, if necessary.

- Provide an accepting environment for the family to express their feelings and fears. Help them recognize that part of their response is normal grief. Assist them in feeling comfortable with their shock, anger, disbelief, denial, depression, or withdrawal.

- Encourage family members to share their feelings and concerns with each other and health care team members frequently. Remind them not to become victims of persistent feelings of guilt or blame.

- Encourage family members to be compassionate and supportive with each other. Reinforce that each individual's adaptation is unique.

- When the family is ready for further knowledge about their infant's treatment and prognosis, help them obtain accurate information.

- Use pictures to help the family visualize the effects of surgical correction of CSF flow.

- Encourage family members to take an active role in the infant's care. Facilitate visits whenever they desire.

- Teach family members how to feed the infant safely. Demonstrate the use of appropriate feeding techniques and equipment. Teach other infant care skills, such as diapering, bathing, and providing cord care.

- Teach family members to suction the infant's oropharynx and nasopharynx gently to help prevent aspiration.

- Emphasize the need to maintain skin integrity on the infant's head. Teach the family to assess for areas of potential breakdown and to reposition the infant frequently. Teach them how to hold the infant safely while supporting the weight of the head.

- Observe for persistent signs of lack of attachment, such as emotional withdrawal from the infant, resistance to infant care, distortion of the prognosis, or fear of taking the infant home.

- Refer the family with attachment difficulties to community agencies as needed.

- Encourage the family to become involved with a support group for parents of infants with congenital defects.

Hyperbilirubinemia

Excessive unconjugated bilirubin in the blood.

NURSING DIAGNOSIS

High risk for injury related to the effects of elevated serum bilirubin level

DESIRED PATIENT OUTCOME

The infant will remain free from injury caused by elevated serum bilirubin level

Outcome measurement criteria

☐ Adequate, early feeding

☐ Meconium stool within 24 hours after birth

☐ Serum bilirubin level within normal limits for the infant's age, size, and ethnic origin

☐ Appropriate response to treatment of elevated serum bilirubin level

☐ Little or no jaundice

Key interventions

• Assess for maternal factors that increase the infant's risk of hyperbilirubinemia, such as infection during pregnancy, diabetes, isoimmunization in an Rh-negative mother, or inadequate prenatal care. Also assess for risk factors in the infant, such as asphyxia or sepsis at birth, low Apgar scores, hypothermia, hypoglycemia, prematurity, low birth weight, cephalhematoma, or soft tissue injuries that caused ecchymosis or hemangiomas.

- Decrease physiologic stressors by rapidly intervening for respiratory difficulty, maintaining a thermally neutral environment, and promptly treating disease.

- Initiate feedings within 4 to 6 hours after birth to promote bowel movements and bilirubin excretion. Observe for and document the presence or absence of meconium stools in the first 24 hours.

- Observe the high-risk infant for the onset of jaundice within the first 24 hours after birth, which may signal pathologic jaundice. Notify the health care professional immediately.

- Monitor the serum bilirubin level according to facility protocol. Report abnormal findings.

- Assess for jaundice by inspecting the infant's sclera and checking the skin color in natural or white light, if possible. To assess the skin, press one thumb or finger over a bony prominence to blanch the skin. Then observe for a golden, orange, or yellow hue before the skin returns to its previous color. To detect early signs of jaundice in a dark-skinned infant, assess the oral mucous membranes and conjunctival sacs.

NURSING DIAGNOSIS
Altered protection related to the effects of phototherapy

DESIRED PATIENT OUTCOME
The infant will remain free from injury cause by phototherapy

Outcome measurement criteria
☐ Absence of corneal irritation or eye drainage
☐ Intact skin
☐ Absence of hyperthermia or hypothermia
☐ Decreased serum bilirubin level

☐ No signs of eye shield pressure around the infant's eyes

Key interventions

- Administer phototherapy as ordered, documenting the equipment used, its distance from the infant, duration of therapy, use of a servo-controlled incubator or open crib, and use of eye protection.

- Protect the infant's eyes from the damaging effects of phototherapy by covering them with patches or specially designed opaque mask devices, such as the Bilimask. Ensure that the infant's eyelids are closed before applying the covering, that the covering is secure and cannot slip off the eyes with head movement, and that it does not put excessive pressure on the eyes.

- Change the eye covering frequently if eye exudate is found on the inside of the cover.

- Place the nude infant under the phototherapy unit. Protect the genitalia with a diaper or a surgical mask that has had its metal noseclip removed.

- Monitor the infant's axillary temperature every 2 to 3 hours. Note hyperthermia or hypothermia and adjust the incubator temperature accordingly.

- Reposition the infant frequently to promote more thorough breakdown of bilirubin.

- Turn off the phototherapy lights and inspect the infant's skin for rash or skin breakdown every 8 hours.

- Promote skin integrity by keeping the perianal area clean and dry. Change soiled diapers and pads as needed.

- Remove the infant from the phototherapy unit and assess the eyes every 4 to 8 hours to detect conjunctivitis. Document findings and notify the health care professional if conjunctivitis occurs.

- Monitor the serum bilirubin level every 4 to 8 hours as ordered. Turn off the phototherapy lights when drawing blood to prevent a false-low reading.

- Monitor the serum bilirubin level every 8 to 12 hours for the first 24 hours after phototherapy is complete, as ordered. Report abnormal findings to the health care professional.

NURSING DIAGNOSIS

High risk for fluid volume deficit related to abnormal fluid loss secondary to phototherapy

DESIRED PATIENT OUTCOME

The infant will display adequate fluid volume during phototherapy

Outcome measurement criteria

☐ Weight loss of no more than 2% per day during photo-therapy

☐ Urine output of at least six wet diapers per day

☐ Fluid intake that equals or exceeds fluid loss

☐ Post-therapy skin turgor that matches pretherapy turgor

☐ Urine specific gravity of 1.001 to 1.020

Key interventions

- Weigh the infant once every 8 hours, particularly noting weight loss of more than 2% of total body weight. Notify the health care professional if significant weight loss occurs.

- Provide feedings every 2 to 4 hours. Offer water between feedings to increase hydration and promote bilirubin excretion.

- Assess the color and quantity of urine and stool output. Weigh diapers to estimate fluid loss. Document fluid intake and urine output.

- Check urine specific gravity once every 8 hours to assess for dehydration.

- Observe for and document other signs of dehydration, such as depressed fontanels, decreased skin turgor, decreased muscle tone, and lethargy. Notify the health care professional if they occur.

- Administer I.V. fluids as prescribed and monitor the insertion site for signs of extravasation.

NURSING DIAGNOSIS

Anxiety (parental) related to lack of knowledge about hyperbilirubinemia and its treatment

DESIRED PATIENT OUTCOME

The parents will display reduced anxiety and increased knowledge of hyperbilirubinemia and its treatment

Outcome measurement criteria

☐ Verbalization of feelings about the infant's condition

☐ Verbalization of an understanding of the treatment plan for hyperbilirubinemia

☐ Participation in the infant's care

☐ Demonstration of attachment behaviors

Key interventions

- Establish a rapport with the infant's parents. Encourage them to discuss feelings, ask questions, and identify concerns.

- Assess the parents' level of knowledge about hyper-bilirubinemia. Offer as much information about the condition as they desire.

- Update the parents about the infant's condition and progress. Help them obtain accurate information about the infant's prognosis.

- Explain that the infant must have an eye covering and be nude during phototherapy.

- Describe the change in appearance of the infant's urine and stool color.

- Remove the infant from the phototherapy unit and remove the eye covering for feedings and interactions with the parents.

- Teach the parents, if needed, how to handle the infant. Encourage them to touch, cuddle, and provide auditory and visual stimulation to promote the infant's emotional well-being.

- Help the parents feed the infant as appropriate. Provide a place for the parents to be alone with the infant. If possible, take the infant to the mother's room for feedings.

- Teach the parents about the need for frequent monitoring of the serum bilirubin level.

- Demonstrate how to assess for jaundice by inspecting blanched skin, mucous membranes, sclerae, and conjunctival sacs.

- Explain the infant's need to consume additional fluid during phototherapy.

- Teach the parents how to safely use prescribed equipment for home phototherapy.

- Observe for persistent signs of lack of attachment, such as emotional withdrawal from the infant, resistance to infant care, distortion of the prognosis, or fear of taking the infant home.

- Refer parents with attachment difficulties to community agencies as needed.

NURSING DIAGNOSIS

Interrupted breast-feeding related to the need for photo-therapy secondary to breast-milk jaundice

DESIRED PATIENT OUTCOME

The mother will reestablish breast-feeding after her infant completes treatment for hyperbilirubinemia

Outcome measurement criteria

☐ Absence of maternal guilt about the infant's condition

☐ Verbalization of an understanding of the infant's jaundice

☐ Regular breast pumping to maintain milk production while the infant receives treatment

☐ Verbalization of resolution to resume breast-feeding

Key interventions

- Assess the mother's understanding of the role of breast milk in jaundice.

- Encourage other family members not to blame the mother for the infant's hyperbilirubinemia. Reassure the mother that she did not cause the infant's condition.

- Provide accurate information about the anticipated treatment, prognosis, and care.

- Answer the mother's questions as they arise during treatment.

- Explore the mother's feelings and plans about resuming breast-feeding.

- Provide information about acquiring a breast pump. As needed, teach the mother how to use the pump and freeze breast milk for later use.

- Help the mother contact support groups that facilitate continuation of breast-feeding, if she desires.

Hypocalcemia

Abnormally low level of serum calcium.

NURSING DIAGNOSIS

High risk for injury related to hypocalcemia

DESIRED PATIENT OUTCOME

The infant will remain free from injury caused by hypocalcemia

Outcome measurement criteria

☐ Appropriate, early nutritional intake

☐ Serum calcium level above 7 mg/dl

☐ Absence of extravasation at I.V. insertion sites

☐ Absence of hypercalcemia

☐ Absence of cardiac arrhythmias

Key interventions

- Assess for maternal factors that increase the infant's risk of hypocalcemia, such as diabetes and hyperparathyroidism. Also assess for infant factors, such as prematurity, small-for-gestational-age status, birth trauma, asphyxia, or exchange transfusion.

- Recognize that hypocalcemia commonly is diagnosed in infants within 48 to 72 hours after birth and 7 days or more after birth.

- Provide a feeding within 2 to 4 hours after birth to help prevent hypocalcemia.

- Advise the parents not to feed the infant cow's milk because it may precipitate late-onset hypocalcemia.

- Observe for signs of hypocalcemia, such as extreme irritability, jitteriness, apnea, cyanosis, abdominal distention, vomiting, abnormal eye movements, unco-ordinated sucking, and high-pitched crying.

- Monitor the serum calcium level. Report abnormal findings to the health care professional and repeat laboratory tests as ordered.

- Maintain a thermally neutral environment to decrease the metabolic demands on the infant.

- Allow for nonnutritive sucking to decrease the infant's activity level.

- Provide maximum rest periods for the infant to prevent tremors or seizures.

- Administer oral calcium supplements as prescribed for the infant with mild hypocalcemia; administer 10% calcium gluconate for one with severe hypocalcemia.

- Administer I.V. push medication slowly, as prescribed, in a well-established I.V. line or through a continuous I.V. delivery system.

- Use extreme caution when administering calcium gluconate. Do not administer I.M. calcium gluconate or administer I.V. calcium gluconate concurrently with a bicarbonate solution or into a scalp vein. (Extravasation into surrounding tissues can cause necrosis.)

- During calcium gluconate administration, monitor the I.V. insertion site continuously for signs of extravasation, such as erythema or edema, and use an electronic monitoring device to assess the infant's heart rate.

- Assess for signs of hypercalcemia, such as vomiting and bradycardia. Discontinue the I.V. infusion and notify the health care professional immediately if the infant's heart rate falls below 100 beats/minute or if vomiting occurs.

- Take seizure precautions for the infant who may have hypercalcemia. Avoid sudden movements of the crib or the infant.

- Monitor the infant's serum calcium level daily as ordered and report findings.

NURSING DIAGNOSIS
Anxiety (parental) related to lack of knowledge about hypocalcemia and its treatment

DESIRED PATIENT OUTCOME
The parents will display reduced anxiety and increased knowledge about hypocalcemia and its treatment

Outcome measurement criteria
☐ Expression of fears, concerns, and feelings about hypocalcemia
☐ Verbalization of an understanding of the treatment plan
☐ Participation in the infant's care
☐ Demonstration of attachment behaviors

Key interventions
- Establish a rapport with the infant's parents. Encourage them to discuss feelings, ask questions, and identify concerns.

- Assess the parents' level of knowledge about hypocalcemia. Provide as much information as the parents desire. Explain that mild, early-onset hypocalcemia usually is temporary and resolves spontaneously.

- Update the parents about the infant's condition and progress.

- Help the parents obtain accurate information about the infant's prognosis.

- Explain the need to minimize stimulation of the infant in the acute phase of moderate or severe hypocalcemia.

- Reassure the parents that, after the acute phase, they will be permitted to hold and cuddle their infant.

- Help the parents feed the infant as appropriate. Provide a place for the parents to be alone with their infant after the acute phase of hypocalcemia.

- Teach the parents about treatment for hypocalcemia and the need for frequent monitoring of the serum calcium level.

- Explain the infant's need for increased rest periods.

- Teach the parents how to prepare and administer dietary calcium supplements if prescribed.

- Observe for persistent signs of lack of attachment, such as emotional withdrawal from the infant, resistance to infant care, distortion of the prognosis, or fear of taking the infant home.

- Refer the family with attachment difficulties to community agencies as needed.

Hypoglycemia

Abnormally low level of serum glucose.

NURSING DIAGNOSIS

High risk for injury related to hypoglycemia

DESIRED PATIENT OUTCOME

The infant will remain free from injury caused by hypoglycemia

Outcome measurement criteria

☐ Adequate, early nutritional intake

☐ Blood glucose level of 45 mg/dl or more by 72 hours after birth

☐ Absence of infiltration at the I.V. insertion site

☐ Absence of more than trace glycosuria

☐ Absence of hypovolemia

☐ Absence of hyperglycemia

Key interventions

• Assess for prenatal factors that increase the infant's risk of hypoglycemia, such as maternal diabetes or sepsis, intrauterine growth retardation, inadequate prenatal care, preeclampsia, eclampsia, or tocolytic treatments. Also assess for factors related to the infant that increase the risk of hypoglycemia, such as small-for-gestational-age or large-for-gestational-age status, prematurity, asphyxia, cold stress, congenital anomalies, sepsis, hypocalcemia, drug withdrawal, or exchange transfusions.

- Provide early feeding (within 2 hours after birth) to help prevent hypoglycemia. For the breast-feeding infant, encourage a feeding; for the bottle-fed infant who is preterm, at risk for hypoglycemia, or suspected to be hypoglycemic, offer 5% dextrose in water (D_5W) orally.

- Maintain a thermally neutral environment to decrease the metabolic demand for glucose.

- Allow for nonnutritive sucking and organize care to allow rest periods to decrease the infant's activity level and energy demands.

- Observe for and document signs of hypoglycemia, such as jitteriness, tremors, jerky movements, seizures, lethargy, decreased muscle tone, rapid irregular respirations, respiratory distress, cyanosis, diaphoresis, apnea, inadequate feeding, vomiting, pallor, or high-pitched crying.

- Test the blood glucose level 1 hour after birth in a full-term appropriate-for-gestational-age infant, immediately after birth in a high-risk infant, or immediately upon detection of signs of hypoglycemia in any infant.

- Monitor the infant's blood glucose level every 4 to 8 hours as ordered during the first 72 hours after birth; for the infant receiving I.V. glucose or oral steroids, monitor the level at least hourly as ordered. To assess the blood glucose level, use a reflectance meter and proper technique. Warm the infant's heel for 5 to 10 seconds before piercing the skin to obtain a blood sample. Repeat the test for the infant with an abnormal blood glucose level to verify the findings. Report abnormal findings to the health care professional.

- Administer I.V. D_5W at 6 to 10 mg/kg/minute as prescribed. Use an infusion pump to regulate the I.V. infusion rate.

- Avoid rapid administration of any I.V. fluids to prevent circulatory overload and hyperglycemia.

- Inspect the I.V. insertion site for signs of infiltration, such as erythema or edema.

- Assess the infant's urine for glycosuria. Report more than trace glycosuria to the health care professional.

- Weigh the infant's diapers to estimate urine output. Notify the health care professional if urine output exceeds 3 ml/kg/hour, which may indicate extreme osmotic diuresis and impending hypovolemia.

NURSING DIAGNOSIS

Anxiety (parental) related to lack of knowledge about hypoglycemia and its treatment

DESIRED PATIENT OUTCOME

The parents will display reduced anxiety and increased knowledge about hypoglycemia and its treatment

Outcome measurement criteria

☐ Expression of fears, concerns, and feelings about hypoglycemia

☐ Verbalization of an understanding of the infant's treatment

☐ Participation in the infant's care

☐ Demonstration of attachment behaviors

Key interventions

- Establish a rapport with the infant's parents. Encourage them to discuss feelings, ask questions, and identify concerns.

- Assess the parents' knowledge about hypoglycemia. Provide as much information as the parents desire.

- Update the parents about the infant's condition and progress.

- Help the parents obtain accurate information about the infant's prognosis.

- Encourage as much physical contact as possible between the parents and infant. Demonstrate safe methods of touching the infant.

- Help the parents feed the infant as appropriate. Provide a place for the parents to be alone with the infant.

- Teach the parents about treatment for hypoglycemia and the need to monitor the blood glucose level frequently. Help the parents realize that repeated heel sticks are required to monitor the blood glucose level accurately.

- Explain the hypoglycemic infant's need for increased rest.

- Observe for persistent signs of lack of attachment, such as emotional withdrawal from the infant, resistance to infant care, distortion of the prognosis, or fear of taking the infant home.

- Refer parents with attachment difficulties to community agencies as needed.

Isoimmune hemolytic anemia

Abnormally rapid destruction of red blood cells caused primarily by Rh or ABO incompatibility in infants.

NURSING DIAGNOSIS

High risk for injury related to the effects of isoimmune hemolytic anemia

DESIRED PATIENT OUTCOME

The infant will remain free from injury caused by isoimmune hemolytic anemia

Outcome measurement criteria

☐ Absence of cardiac arrhythmias

☐ Absence of hyperthermia or hypothermia

☐ Absence of signs of hypocalcemia

☐ Decreased serum bilirubin level by approximately 50% after the exchange transfusion

Key interventions

• Assess for factors that increase the infant's risk of isoimmune hemolytic anemia, such as an Rh-negative mother who was not treated with $Rh_o(D)$ immune globulin (RhoGAM) after an abortion, ectopic pregnancy, or amniocentesis; within 72 hours after delivery of a previous Rh-positive infant; or at 28 weeks' gestation with this infant. Additional risk factors include an Rh-negative mother who has received a transfusion of Rh-positive blood, delivered an infant who required an exchange transfusion, obtained inadequate prenatal care, or has type O blood.

- Observe the infant for the onset of jaundice within 24 hours after birth. If jaundice occurs, notify the health care professional and evaluate the infant's serum bilirubin level as ordered.

- Obtain typed and cross-matched blood as ordered.

- Ensure that the infant receives nothing by mouth for 3 to 4 hours before the exchange transfusion, or empty the stomach with nasogastric suction as ordered.

- Gather the necessary equipment at the bedside. Place monitors on the infant and keep resuscitation equipment at hand. Restrain the infant as needed and as ordered.

- Assist the health care professional with the exchange transfusion as needed. During and after the transfusion, monitor and document the infant's vital signs according to facility protocol. Also document the amount of blood given and withdrawn and the amount and type of medication administered.

- Use blankets or a radiant warmer to maintain optimum body temperature for the infant.

- Assess the transfusion site frequently for bleeding, redness, and swelling after the transfusion.

- Report the serum bilirubin level as ordered. Expect the post-transfusion level to be about 50% of the pretransfusion level.

- Observe for signs of complications, such as metabolic acidosis, hypothermia, circulatory overload, electrolyte imbalance, air embolism, arrhythmias, infection, and hypoglycemia.

- Resume feedings as soon as possible after the exchange transfusion. Gavage feed the infant as ordered.

- Have 2 more units of blood typed and cross-matched after the initial transfusion is complete in case additional transfusions become necessary.

NURSING DIAGNOSIS

Altered family processes related to lack of knowledge about isoimmune hemolytic anemia and interruption of parent-infant attachment

DESIRED PATIENT OUTCOME

The family will display increased knowledge about isoimmune hemolytic anemia and will demonstrate attachment behaviors

Outcome measurement criteria

☐ Expression of feelings about the infant's condition

☐ Expression of mutual support among family members

☐ Verbalization of an understanding of the infant's treatment plan

☐ Participation in the infant's care

☐ Demonstration of attachment behaviors

Key interventions

• Establish a rapport with the infant's family. Encourage family members to discuss feelings, ask questions, and identify concerns.

• Assess the family's knowledge of isoimmune hemolytic anemia. Provide as much information as the family desires.

• Update the family frequently about the infant's condition and progress.

• Encourage family members to visit and call the nursery.

• Help the family obtain accurate information about the infant's prognosis.

• Emphasize the positive aspects of the infant.

- Teach family members, if needed, how to handle the infant. Encourage them to touch, cuddle, and provide auditory and visual stimulation to promote the infant's emotional well-being.

- Help family members feed the infant as appropriate. Provide a place for them to be alone with the infant.

- Observe for persistent signs of lack of attachment, such as emotional withdrawal from the infant, resistance to infant care, distortion of the prognosis, or fear of taking the infant home.

- Refer the family with attachment difficulties to community agencies as needed.

Meconium aspiration syndrome

Respiratory disease caused by inhalation of meconium or meconium-stained amniotic fluid into the bronchial tree.

NURSING DIAGNOSIS

Impaired gas exchange related to meconium aspirate in the respiratory tract

DESIRED PATIENT OUTCOME

The infant will exhibit adequate ventilation and gas exchange to support life

Outcome measurement criteria

☐ Respiratory rate of 30 to 60 breaths/minute

☐ Absence of cyanosis or apneic episodes

☐ Normal breath sounds on auscultation

☐ Pulse oximetry value of more than 95%

☐ Capillary refill time of less than 4 seconds

☐ Age-appropriate arterial blood gas (ABG) levels

Key interventions

• Assess for factors that increase the infant's risk of meconium aspiration syndrome (MAS), such as prolonged labor; maternal illness; preterm, post-term, breech, or cesarean delivery; small-for-gestational-age status; fetal distress during labor; presence of meconium-stained amniotic fluid; intrauterine growth retardation; or low Apgar scores. Notify the health care professional if meconium-stained amniotic fluid or other risk factors exist.

- Suction the nares, mouth, and pharynx before delivery of the infant's thorax; suction again after delivery is complete.

- Assist with visualization of the vocal folds and suctioning of the trachea.

- Place the infant in a thermally neutral environment to decrease the metabolic demand.

- Assess the infant's respiratory rate, depth, and effort. Observe for and report signs of respiratory distress, such as episodes of apnea, nasal flaring, grunting, and accessory muscle use.

- Auscultate the lungs to detect adventitious breath sounds. Particularly note signs of respiratory deterioration, such as basilar crackles and decreased breath sounds.

- Observe the infant for increasing generalized cyanosis and the onset of circumoral pallor or cyanosis.

- Monitor and document the pulse oximetry value. Notify the health care professional of decreasing values.

- Administer oxygen as ordered; assist with intubation and mechanical ventilation as needed.

- Use apnea and cardiac monitors for ongoing evaluations.

- Administer I.V. fluids and medications as prescribed to correct alkalosis, increase fluid volume, and decrease the metabolic demand for oxygen. Administer prophylactic antibiotics as prescribed.

- Ensure that the respiratory support equipment is patent.

- Report ABG levels as ordered. Be alert for increasing hypoxia, hypercapnia, and acidosis.

- Provide chest physiotherapy as ordered to promote mobilization of pulmonary secretions.

NURSING DIAGNOSIS

High risk for infection related to invasive monitors used during the treatment of MAS

DESIRED PATIENT OUTCOME

The infant will display no signs or symptoms of infection during the treatment of MAS

Outcome measurement criteria

☐ Rectal temperature of 97.7° to 99.5° F (36.5° to 37.5° C)

☐ Absence of tachypnea or tachycardia

☐ Normal breath sounds on auscultation

☐ White blood cell (WBC) count within normal limits

☐ Absence of signs of infection at the I.V. insertion site

Key interventions

- Monitor the infant's vital signs and graph the findings.

- Observe for trends in vital signs that may indicate the onset of infection, such as fever, tachypnea, and tachycardia. Notify the health care professional if such signs occur.

- Auscultate the infant's lungs, noting any deterioration in breath sounds.

- Review the infant's WBC count and report an elevated count.

- Use strict aseptic or sterile technique when caring for the infant, especially when changing the tubing on respiratory and I.V. administration equipment.

- Assess for signs of local infection at the I.V. insertion site. Observe for interrupted skin integrity at sites where monitors have been attached.

- Administer prophylactic antibiotics as prescribed.

Nursing Diagnosis

Altered family processes related to lack of knowledge about MAS and interruption of parent-infant attachment

DESIRED PATIENT OUTCOME

The family will display increased knowledge about MAS and will demonstrate appropriate attachment behaviors

Outcome measurement criteria

☐ Expression of feelings about the infant's condition

☐ Expression of mutual support among family members

☐ Verbalization of an understanding of the infant's treatment plan

☐ Participation in the infant's care

☐ Demonstration of attachment behaviors

Key interventions

• Establish a rapport with the infant's family. Encourage family members to discuss feelings, ask questions, and identify concerns.

• Assess the family's knowledge of MAS. Provide as much information as the family desires.

• Update the family frequently about the infant's condition and progress.

• Encourage family members to visit and call the nursery.

• Help the family obtain accurate information about the infant's prognosis.

• Emphasize the positive aspects of the infant.

• Teach family members, if needed, how to provide gentle auditory and visual stimulation to promote the infant's emotional well-being. Explain the infant's need for minimal physical stimulation and reassure them that they can cuddle and hold the infant after recovery from the acute phase.

- Help family members feed the infant as appropriate. Provide a place for them to be alone with the infant.

- Observe for persistent signs of lack of attachment, such as emotional withdrawal from the infant, resistance to infant care, distortion of the prognosis, or fear of taking the infant home.

- Refer the family with attachment difficulties to community agencies as needed.

Necrotizing enterocolitis

Acute inflammation of the bowel that causes necrosis of the GI mucosa.

NURSING DIAGNOSIS

High risk for injury related to the progression of necrosis

DESIRED PATIENT OUTCOME

The infant will remain free from bowel injury caused by the progression of necrosis

Outcome measurement criteria

☐ Bowel sounds in all quadrants

☐ Absence of GI bleeding

☐ Absence of abdominal rigidity or increasing abdominal girth

☐ Absence of bile-colored vomitus

☐ Absence of signs of septic shock

Key interventions

• Assess for and document bowel sounds in the infant with necrotizing enterocolitis (NEC). Initially, bowel sounds may be hyperactive. During treatment of the acute phase, they may be absent. When feedings resume, they should recur.

• Test for occult blood in the stool. Observe the stool color; dark brown or red streaks may indicate GI bleeding.

• Provide continuous gastric decompression by inserting a nasogastric tube as ordered.

- Measure and document the infant's abdominal girth every 4 to 8 hours. Be aware that increasing abdominal girth is an ominous sign of the progression of necrosis.
- Gently palpate the abdomen, noting increased rigidity.
- Inspect vomitus to detect bile or blood.
- Observe for signs of bleeding, such as petechiae, ecchymosis, prolonged capillary refill time, and decreased hemoglobin and hematocrit values; also assess for signs of shock, such as widening pulse pressure, tachycardia, apnea, bradypnea, and hypothermia.
- Report signs of deterioration in the infant's condition.
- Administer antibiotics as prescribed. Administer oxygen and initiate life-support techniques as ordered.

NURSING DIAGNOSIS

Fluid volume deficit related to nothing-by-mouth status, the need for bowel rest, and abnormal fluid loss through vomiting and diarrhea

DESIRED PATIENT OUTCOME

The infant will display adequate fluid volume

Outcome measurement criteria

☐ Absence of signs of dehydration

☐ Absence of tachycardia

☐ Absence of vomiting or diarrhea

☐ Urine specific gravity of 1.001 to 1.020

☐ Weight loss of no more than 2% per day

☐ Stable weight after initial recovery of birth weight

☐ Serum electrolyte levels within normal limits

Key interventions

- Assess for and report signs of dehydration, such as decreased skin turgor, increased tachycardia, dry mucous membranes, and depressed fontanels.

- Record the infant's fluid intake and urine output. Weigh the infant's diapers to measure urine output accurately. Estimate the volume of any vomiting or diarrhea; include these estimates in the intake and output records.

- Measure the urine specific gravity as ordered, being alert for increasing specific gravity.

- Weigh the infant daily and record findings. Analyze the records for persistent weight loss.

- Notify the health care professional if the infant shows signs of dehydration or abnormal fluid loss.

- Administer I.V. fluids and total parenteral nutrition (TPN) as prescribed to increase the fluid volume and meet dietary needs.

- Monitor laboratory test results as ordered and report abnormal findings. Be alert for alkalosis or hyperkalemia, which may result from GI obstruction.

NURSING DIAGNOSIS

High risk for altered nutrition: less than body requirements, related to treatment of NEC

DESIRED PATIENT OUTCOME

The infant will obtain sufficient nutrients to support recovery and growth

Outcome measurement criteria

☐ Weight gain of 0.5 to 1.1 oz (15 to 30 g) per day

☐ Intake of 110 to 150 calories/kg/day

☐ Serum glucose level of 45 to 90 mg/dl

Key interventions

- Weigh the infant at the same time every day, using the same scale. Document weight changes so that the infant's progress can be tracked easily.

- Calculate caloric and fluid needs every day based on the infant's current weight.

- Monitor the infant's blood glucose level to determine if sufficient energy is available to meet metabolic demands.

- Administer I.V. fluids that contain glucose and TPN as prescribed.

- Notify the health care professional of loss of more than 2% of body weight in 24 hours.

NURSING DIAGNOSIS

Altered family processes related to lack of knowledge about NEC and interruption of parent-infant attachment

DESIRED PATIENT OUTCOME

The family will display increased knowledge about NEC and will demonstrate attachment behaviors

Outcome measurement criteria

- ☐ Expression of feelings about the infant's condition
- ☐ Expression of mutual support among family members
- ☐ Verbalization of an understanding of the infant's treatment plan
- ☐ Participation in the infant's care
- ☐ Demonstration of attachment behaviors

Key interventions

- Establish a rapport with the infant's family. Encourage family members to discuss feelings, ask questions, and identify concerns.

- Assess the family's knowledge of NEC. Provide as much information as the family desires.

- Update the family frequently about the infant's condition and progress.

- Encourage family members to visit and call the nursery.

- Help the family obtain accurate information about the infant's prognosis.

- Emphasize the positive aspects of the infant.

- Teach family members about interventions for short-bowel syndrome, including temporary colostomy. Reassure them that they can learn to provide colostomy care.

- Teach family members, if needed, how to handle the infant. Encourage gentle stroking and quiet auditory stimulation to promote the infant's emotional well-being.

- Explain the infant's need for minimal physical stimulation during the acute phase. Reassure family members that they may cuddle and hold the infant after the initial recovery from infection. Provide a place for them to be alone with the infant.

- Observe for persistent signs of lack of attachment, such as emotional withdrawal from the infant, resistance to infant care, distortion of the prognosis, or fear of taking the infant home.

- Refer the family with attachment difficulties to community agencies as needed.

Peripheral nervous system injury

Peripheral nerve damage during birth that causes transient or permanent paralysis.

NURSING DIAGNOSIS
High risk for injury related to birth trauma

DESIRED PATIENT OUTCOME
The infant will remain free from injury caused by peripheral nervous system injury

Outcome measurement criteria
☐ Oral intake within normal limits
☐ Absence of permanent eye damage
☐ Absence of permanent paralysis

Key interventions
- Assess for factors that increase the infant's risk of peripheral nerve injury, such as forceps-assisted delivery, cephalopelvic disproportion, macrosomia, dystocia, and maternal diabetes.

- Immediately after birth, assess for asymmetrical arm and leg movements and facial muscles and difficulty breathing. Notify the health care professional if such signs occur.

- For upper brachial plexus injury or Erb-Duchenne paralysis, stabilize the affected arm with 90-degree abduction, external shoulder rotation, 90-degree elbow flexion, forearm supination, and slight wrist dorsiflexion. To enhance stabilization, apply a light dressing or tape around the affected forearm and wrist, with edges approximately 2" (5 cm) from the infant; safety-pin these edges to the sheet to position the arm appropriately.

- For facial paralysis, administer artificial tears as prescribed every 2 to 4 hours.

- Use a soft nipple with a medium to large hole to promote feeding in a bottle-fed infant. Show the mother how to compress the areola and place the nipple far back in the mouth for the breast-fed infant. If sucking does not allow sufficient fluid intake, gavage-feed the infant as ordered.

- For phrenic nerve injury, assist with resuscitation at birth and with mechanical ventilation.

NURSING DIAGNOSIS

Anxiety (parental) related to disappointment with the infant's appearance, uncertainty about the prognosis, and lack of knowledge about the infant's care

DESIRED PATIENT OUTCOME

The parents will display reduced anxiety and will participate effectively in the infant's care

Outcome measurement criteria

☐ Expression of feelings about the condition and increased comfort with the infant

☐ Verbalization of an understanding of the treatment and prognosis for peripheral nervous system injury

☐ Demonstration of appropriate infant care techniques

☐ Demonstration of attachment behaviors

Key interventions

- Establish a supportive relationship with the parents. Encourage them to express their concerns, fears, disappointments, joys, and other feelings.

- Help the parents obtain accurate information about the treatment plan and prognosis.

- Encourage the parents to ask questions whenever they desire.

- Demonstrate feeding and care techniques appropriate to the infant's specific condition. Give the parents time to practice these techniques before the infant is discharged.

- Teach the parents how to position the affected arm or leg for the infant with Erb-Duchenne's paralysis.

- Teach the parents to avoid excessive stimulation of the affected arm or leg for the first 10 days after birth. After that, instruct them to gently massage the arm or leg and perform gentle range-of-motion exercises daily to avoid contractures.

- Emphasize the importance of vigilant care to promote full recovery from peripheral nerve injury. Stress the need for timely follow-up examinations with the health care professional.

- Teach the parents, if needed, how to handle the infant. Encourage them to touch, cuddle, and provide auditory and visual stimulation to promote the infant's emotional well-being.

- Observe for persistent signs of lack of attachment, such as emotional withdrawal from the infant, resistance to infant care, distortion of the prognosis, or fear of taking the infant home.

- Refer the family with attachment difficulties to community agencies as needed.

Respiratory distress syndrome

Respiratory condition often associated with prematurity that causes inappropriate gas exchange at the alveolar level.

NURSING DIAGNOSIS

Impaired gas exchange related to inadequate lung surfactant and decreased alveolar perfusion secondary to prematurity

DESIRED PATIENT OUTCOME

The infant will demonstrate adequate gas exchange to support life

Outcome measurement criteria

☐ Respiratory rate of 30 to 60 breaths/minute

☐ Absence of signs of respiratory distress

☐ Absence of cyanosis

☐ Normal breath sounds on auscultation

☐ Pulse oximetry value of more than 95%

☐ Capillary refill time of less than 4 seconds

☐ Arterial blood gas levels within normal ranges

Key interventions

- Assess for factors that increase the infant's risk of respiratory distress syndrome (RDS), such as prematurity, lecithin-sphingomyelin ratio of less than 2:1, asphyxia or resuscitation at birth, maternal diabetes, placental bleeding, or signs of respiratory distress.

- Keep resuscitation equipment at the infant's bedside.

- Place the infant in a thermally neutral environment to decrease the metabolic demand.

- Assess the respiratory rate, depth, and effort. Observe for signs of respiratory distress, such as apneic episodes, nasal flaring, grunting, and accessory muscle use. Document findings and notify the health care professional immediately if any of these signs increase.

- Inspect the infant for increasing generalized cyanosis and the onset of circumoral pallor or mottling.

- Auscultate the lungs to detect decreasing breath sounds or adventitious breath sounds, such as basilar crackles.

- Monitor the infant's pulse oximetry value. Document findings and report the onset of deterioration.

- Administer oxygen as ordered. Assist with intubation and mechanical ventilation as needed.

- Use apnea and cardiac monitors to help assess the infant.

- Administer I.V. fluids and medications as prescribed to decrease acidosis, increase fluid volume, and decrease the metabolic demand for oxygen.

- Ensure the patency of respiratory support equipment.

- Report laboratory test results, as ordered. Be alert for increasing hypoxia, hypercapnia, or acidosis.

NURSING DIAGNOSIS

Activity intolerance related to inadequate pulmonary function secondary to prematurity

DESIRED PATIENT OUTCOME

The infant will experience minimal energy expenditure during activities and will demonstrate improved tolerance of activity

Outcome measurement criteria

☐ Vital signs within normal limits

☐ Achievement of adequate sleep and rest

☐ Absence of cyanosis or apneic episodes during activity

Key interventions

• Minimize physical stimulation of the infant with RDS to help decrease the metabolic demand for oxygen.

• Provide a restful, thermally neutral environment.

• Cluster nursing interventions to allow increased rest periods.

• Anticipate the infant's needs so that discomfort and hunger are addressed before increased activity occurs.

• Feed the infant by the I.V., gavage, or continuous nasogastric method to minimize energy expenditure.

• Maintain the patency of I.V. lines and monitors to avoid having to restart invasive devices, which could further stress the infant.

• Do not allow the infant to be touched, except when direct care is provided or when the family visits. When the infant must be handled, move gently, slowly, and purposefully.

• Administer a sedative as prescribed to decrease activity in an infant who has difficulty with gas exchange during activity.

NURSING DIAGNOSIS

High risk for altered nutrition: less than body requirements, related to treatment for RDS

DESIRED PATIENT OUTCOME

The infant will obtain sufficient nutrients to support recovery and growth

Outcome measurement criteria

☐ Weight gain of 0.5 to 1.1 oz (15 to 30 g) per day

☐ Intake of 110 to 150 calories/kg/day

☐ Serum glucose level of 45 to 90 mg/dl

Key interventions

• Weigh the infant at the same time every day, using the same scale. Document weight changes so that the infant's progress can be tracked easily.

• Calculate caloric and fluid needs every day based on the infant's current weight.

• Monitor the infant's blood glucose level to determine if sufficient energy is available to meet metabolic demands.

• Administer I.V. fluids that contain glucose and provide total parenteral nutrition as prescribed.

• Notify the health care professional of a loss of more than 2% of body weight in 24 hours.

NURSING DIAGNOSIS

High risk for infection related to the use of invasive monitors during treatment for RDS

DESIRED PATIENT OUTCOME

The infant will display no signs or symptoms of infection during treatment

Outcome measurement criteria

☐ Rectal temperature of 97.7° to 99.5° F (36.5° to 37.5° C)

☐ Absence of tachypnea or tachycardia

☐ Normal breath sounds on auscultation

☐ White blood cell (WBC) count within normal limits

☐ Absence of signs of infection at the I.V. insertion site

Key interventions

- Monitor the infant's vital signs and graph the findings.

- Observe for trends in vital signs that may indicate the onset of infection, such as fever, tachypnea, and tachycardia. Notify the health care professional if such signs occur.

- Auscultate the infant's lungs, noting any deterioration in breath sounds.

- Review the infant's WBC count and report an elevated count.

- Use strict aseptic or sterile technique when caring for the infant, especially when changing the tubing on respiratory and I.V. administration equipment.

- Assess for signs of local infection at the I.V. insertion site. Observe for interrupted skin integrity at sites where monitors have been attached.

- Administer prophylactic antibiotics as prescribed.

NURSING DIAGNOSIS

Altered family processes related to lack of knowledge about RDS and interruption of parent-infant attachment

DESIRED PATIENT OUTCOME

The family will display increased knowledge about RDS and will demonstrate attachment behaviors

Outcome measurement criteria

☐ Expression of feelings about the infant's condition

☐ Expression of mutual support among family members

☐ Verbalization of an understanding of the infant's treatment plan

☐ Participation in the infant's care

☐ Demonstration of attachment behaviors

Key interventions

• Establish a rapport with the infant's family. Encourage family members to discuss feelings, ask questions, and identify concerns.

• Assess the family's knowledge of RDS. Provide as much information as the family desires.

• Update the family frequently about the infant's condition and progress.

• Encourage family members to visit and call the nursery.

• Help the family obtain accurate information about the infant's prognosis.

• Emphasize the positive aspects of the infant.

• Teach family members how to handle the infant, if needed. Encourage gentle stroking and quiet auditory stimulation to promote the infant's emotional well-being. Explain the infant's need for minimal physical stimulation; reassure family members that they may cuddle and hold the infant after recovery from the acute phase.

• Help family members feed the infant as appropriate. Provide a place for them to be alone with the infant.

• Observe for persistent signs of lack of attachment, such as emotional withdrawal from the infant, resistance to infant care, distortion of the prognosis, or fear of taking the infant home.

• Refer the family with attachment difficulties to community agencies as needed.

Sepsis neonatorum

Infectious disease in infants that occurs before, during, or after birth, especially in premature infants.

NURSING DIAGNOSIS

Altered protection related to the presence of infectious organisms and the infant's immature immune system

DESIRED PATIENT OUTCOME

The infant will remain free from injury caused by sepsis neonatorum

Outcome measurement criteria

☐ Respiratory rate of 30 to 60 breaths/minute

☐ Heart rate of 110 to 160 beats/minute

☐ Rectal temperature of 97.7° to 99.5° F (36.5° to 37.5° C)

☐ White blood cell (WBC) count within normal limits

☐ Bilirubin level within normal limits

☐ Blood glucose level within normal limits

Key interventions

• Assess for prenatal factors that increase the infant's risk of sepsis neonatorum, such as inadequate prenatal care; maternal illness, TORCH infection, sexually transmitted disease, or bleeding disorder; or premature rupture of membranes. Be alert for intrapartal risk factors, such as toxemia, fetal distress, asphyxia, and chorioamnionitis. Also check for risk factors related to the infant, such as prematurity, aseptic delivery, meconium aspiration, small-for-gestational-age status, or presence of a congenital anomaly or of interrupted skin integrity caused by monitors.

- Decrease the infant's risk of contracting a nosocomial infection by washing hands thoroughly, observing appropriate isolation precautions, using appropriate aseptic or sterile technique, and avoiding overcrowding in the nursery.

- Assess and document the infant's vital signs. Particularly note signs of infection, such as tachycardia; hyperthermia; tachypnea, apnea, or irregular respirations; hypotension; or pale or mottled skin.

- Use a servo-controlled incubator to keep the infant's temperature within normal limits.

- Monitor the infant for changes in feeding or consistently poor feeding, vomiting, diarrhea, or failure to digest feedings, which may signal sepsis neonatorum.

- Note changes in the infant's activity and comfort level. Hypotonia or hypertonia, lethargy, irritability, high-pitched crying, abnormal eye movements, and seizures may signal sepsis neonatorum.

- Inspect the infant's skin for irritation, rash, redness, or edema.

- Monitor the infant's laboratory test results, as ordered. Signs of sepsis neonatorum may include a WBC count under $5,000/mm^3$ or over $25,000/mm^3$; hyperbilirubinemia; and an elevated blood glucose level.

- Report findings that suggest sepsis neonatorum.

- Obtain specimens for culture and sensitivity testing, and prepare the infant for X-rays as ordered.

- Administer I.V. fluids and antibiotics as prescribed.

- Use an electronic device to constantly monitor the infant at risk for sepsis neonatorum.

NURSING DIAGNOSIS

Impaired gas exchange related to the physiologic effects of sepsis neonatorum

DESIRED PATIENT OUTCOME

The infant will display adequate ventilation and gas exchange to support life

Outcome measurement criteria

- ☐ Respiratory rate of 30 to 60 breaths/minute
- ☐ Heart rate of 110 to 160 beats/minute
- ☐ Absence of cyanosis or apneic episodes
- ☐ Capillary refill time of less than 4 seconds
- ☐ Normal breath sounds on auscultation
- ☐ Age-appropriate arterial blood gas (ABG) levels
- ☐ Pulse oximetry value of more than 95%

Key interventions

- Monitor the infant for signs of decreased ventilation. Document tachypnea, apnea, or tachycardia.
- Inspect the infant for increasing cyanosis or circumoral pallor.
- Assess the capillary refill time and record the results.
- Auscultate the lungs to detect adventitious breath sounds.
- Notify the health care professional of findings that suggest inadequate ventilation and gas exchange.
- Obtain and report ABG and pulse oximetry values as ordered.
- Administer oxygen as ordered.
- Maintain resuscitation equipment at the infant's bedside.

NURSING DIAGNOSIS

High risk for fluid volume deficit related to the physiologic effects of sepsis neonatorum

DESIRED PATIENT OUTCOME

The infant will display adequate fluid volume to support life

Outcome measurement criteria

- ☐ Urine output of at least 2 ml/kg/hour
- ☐ Urine specific gravity of 1.001 to 1.020
- ☐ Absence of signs of dehydration
- ☐ Blood urea nitrogen (BUN), creatinine, and serum electrolyte levels within normal limits
- ☐ Absence of vomiting or diarrhea

Key interventions

- Maintain a thermally neutral environment to decrease insensible fluid loss.

- Monitor and record the infant's fluid intake and urine output hourly. Weigh diapers to measure urine output accurately. Document the frequency and volume of vomiting and diarrhea and include these amounts in the output totals. Calculate the need for fluid replacement based on total intake and output information.

- Assess the infant's urine specific gravity. Note increasing specific gravity, which may indicate dehydration.

- Assess for other signs of dehydration, including depressed fontanels, lethargy, decreased skin turgor, and dry mucous membranes.

- Notify the health care professional of the infant's fluid volume status as ordered.

- Monitor the infant's renal function by checking BUN and creatinine levels. Monitor serum electrolyte levels to detect any imbalances. Report laboratory test results.
- Administer I.V. fluids, electrolytes, and total parenteral nutrition as prescribed.

NURSING DIAGNOSIS

Altered family processes related to lack of knowledge about sepsis neonatorum and interruption of parent-infant attachment

DESIRED PATIENT OUTCOME

The family will display increased knowledge about sepsis neonatorum and will demonstrate attachment behaviors

Outcome measurement criteria

☐ Expression of feelings about the infant's condition

☐ Expression of mutual support among family members

☐ Verbalization of an understanding of the infant's treatment plan

☐ Participation in the infant's care

☐ Demonstration of attachment behaviors

Key interventions

- Establish a rapport with the infant's family. Encourage family members to discuss feelings, ask questions, and identify concerns.
- Assess the family's knowledge of sepsis neonatorum. Provide as much information as the family desires.
- Update the family frequently about the infant's condition and progress.
- Encourage family members to visit and call the nursery.

- Help the family obtain accurate information about the infant's prognosis.

- Emphasize the positive aspects of the infant.

- Teach family members how to handle the infant, if needed. Encourage gentle stroking and quiet auditory stimulation to promote the infant's emotional well-being. Explain the infant's need for minimal physical stimulation; reassure family members that they may cuddle and hold the infant after recovery from the acute phase.

- Teach the family how to decrease the risk of infection by maintaining a clean environment and washing the hands frequently.

- Help family members feed the infant as appropriate. Provide a place for them to be alone with the infant.

- Observe for persistent signs of lack of attachment, such as emotional withdrawal from the infant, resistance to infant care, distortion of the prognosis, or fear of taking the infant home.

- Refer the family with attachment difficulties to community agencies as needed.

Skeletal injury

Damage to the infant's skeleton during birth.

NURSING DIAGNOSIS

Pain related to skeletal injury and tissue trauma

DESIRED PATIENT OUTCOME

The infant will display minimal signs of pain caused by skeletal injury or tissue trauma

Outcome measurement criteria

☐ Demonstration of pain relief

☐ Absence of increased edema, hematoma, or skin discoloration

☐ Little or no mobility restrictions

Key interventions

• Assess for factors that increase the infant's risk of skeletal injury, such as forceps-assisted delivery, breech presentation, cephalopelvic disproportion, macrosomia, maternal diabetes, dystocia, or precipitous labor and delivery.

• Observe for edema, ecchymosis, lesions, abrasions, hematomas, and petechiae. If any of these are present, thoroughly examine the surrounding area for skeletal injury.

• Be alert for asymmetry or abnormal movement of the arms, legs, or facial features, which indicate the need for further evaluation.

• Palpate for crepitus over a suspected skeletal fracture. Document findings.

- Notify the health care professional of findings that suggest skeletal injury. Begin treatments as ordered.

- Treat a clavicular fracture with gentle handling to minimize pain. Teach family members to handle the infant gently and to keep the affected area properly aligned.

- Assist with application of an immobilization device for a fractured humerus or femur, as needed. Teach the family how to maintain the sling, splint, or other device.

- For an uncomplicated linear skull fracture, use gentle handling during treatment.

- Observe for increased edema, erythema, ecchymosis, crepitus, decreased peripheral circulation, or behavior changes, which may signal increasing damage or bleeding at the injury site. Notify the health care professional if these signs occur.

- Inform the family that healing of fractures typically takes 3 to 4 weeks.

- Teach the family how to bathe, feed, and clothe the infant carefully while supporting the injured area to decrease pain and promote healing.

- Observe for jaundice in the infant with significant ecchymosis. Inform the family that jaundice may develop as the ecchymosis resolves. Teach them how to assess for jaundice by gently blanching the skin or assessing the mucous membranes.

- Arrange for follow-up visits as ordered.

Soft tissue injury

Damage to the infant's soft tissue during delivery, which may cause erythema, ecchymosis, edema, petechiae, abrasions, or lacerations.

NURSING DIAGNOSIS

Anxiety (parental) related to lack of knowledge about soft tissue injury

DESIRED PATIENT OUTCOME

The parents will display reduced anxiety and increased knowledge about soft tissue injury

Outcome measurement criteria

☐ Verbalization of an understanding of the cause of soft tissue injury

☐ Verbalization of an understanding of the management and prognosis for soft tissue injury

☐ Demonstration of attachment behaviors

Key interventions

• Teach the parents that soft tissue injuries are common in infants. Explain the cause of the infant's injury (if known), such as breech or face presentation, forceps use, cephalopelvic disproportion, or a nuchal cord.

• Reassure the parents that soft tissue injuries typically are benign and resolve with no residual problems. Explain that edema, ecchymosis, petechiae, abrasions, and lacerations usually subside with minimal intervention during the first week after delivery.

- Encourage the parents not to be afraid to touch their infant because of the soft tissue injury. Demonstrate nurturing behaviors as needed.

- Encourage the parents to discuss feelings about the infant's appearance. Explain that it is normal for them to feel disappointed.

- Keep the soft tissue injury clean, and apply ointments and medications as prescribed to maintain skin integrity and decrease the risk of infection. Teach the parents about required care.

- Observe for persistent signs of lack of attachment, such as emotional withdrawal from the infant, resistance to infant care, distortion of the prognosis, or fear of taking the infant home.

- Refer the family with attachment difficulties to community agencies as needed.

Spina bifida

Congenital defect in closure of the vertebral column, which typically allows the meninges or spinal cord to protrude.

NURSING DIAGNOSIS

High risk for infection related to altered skin integrity over the protruding sac or over bony prominences

DESIRED PATIENT OUTCOME

The infant will show no signs or symptoms of infection

Outcome measurement criteria

☐ Absence of increased restlessness and irritability

☐ Absence of pressure ulcers on bony prominences

☐ Absence of skin breakdown over meningocele or myelomeningocele

☐ Rectal temperature of 97.7° to 99.5° F (36.5° to 37.5° C)

☐ Respiratory rate of 30 to 60 breaths/minute

☐ Heart rate of 120 to 160 beats/minute

☐ White blood cell (WBC) count within normal limits

Key interventions

• Assess the infant's behavior patterns for signs of physiologic distress or infection, such as increased irritability, crying, or restlessness.

• Place the infant in a prone position to protect the protruding sac. If possible, periodically place the infant in a modified side-lying position with small pillows for support. Change or modify the infant's position as much as possible every 2 hours.

- Protect the sac from contamination and irritants by covering it with a sterile dressing moistened with sterile saline and then covering the dressing with plastic wrap. Change the dressing and plastic wrap every 2 hours as ordered.

- Remove stool promptly and apply a moisture barrier around the anus as ordered to prevent skin breakdown.

- Assess the skin over bony prominences for signs of breakdown. Keep the infant on clean, dry, soft linens and use a sheepskin or egg-crate mattress to protect against pressure ulcers.

- Gently massage the skin over bony prominences and apply lotion or ointment as ordered.

- Handle the infant carefully to avoid injury to the sac. Hold the infant prone on the lap when burping or cuddling.

- Dress the infant carefully to avoid contact between the clothing and the sac. If necessary, avoid clothing the infant and secure the diapers loosely or place them under the infant to avoid irritating the sac.

- Observe for and document any leakage or rupture of the sac. Notify the health care professional immediately.

- Monitor and document the infant's temperature and respiratory and heart rates every 4 hours. Rising temperature, tachypnea, or tachycardia may signal the onset of infection.

- Review the infant's WBC count and report any elevation.

- Administer antibiotics as prescribed.

NURSING DIAGNOSIS

Ineffective thermoregulation related to an open lesion on the spinal column

DESIRED PATIENT OUTCOME

The infant will maintain a temperature within normal limits

Outcome measurement criteria

☐ Rectal temperature of 97.7° to 99.5° F (36.5° to 37.5° C)

☐ Absence of tachypnea

☐ Absence of cyanosis or deepening acrocyanosis

Key interventions

- Assess the infant's temperature at birth, hourly until it is stable, and then every 4 hours.

- Keep the infant in an incubator with a servo-control unit to provide a thermally neutral environment.

- Keep the infant's environment dry and avoid prolonged exposure to moist bedding.

- Use warm sterile saline to moisten the dressing for the sac. Apply the warm dressing and cover it with plastic wrap to decrease evaporative heat loss.

- Observe and document the respiratory rate. Be alert for tachypnea, which may result from an increased oxygen demand.

- Observe for generalized cyanosis or increasing acro-cyanosis, which may signal an increase in the metabolic demand caused by thermogenesis. Assess the acrocyano-tic infant's mucous membranes to evaluate cyanosis or acrocyanosis more accurately.

- If a thermistor probe is used to assess skin temperature, periodically verify readings by taking an axillary tem-perature.

NURSING DIAGNOSIS

Ineffective family coping: compromised, related to grief over the loss of the idealized infant and guilt, fear, anxiety, and lack of knowledge about spina bifida

DESIRED PATIENT OUTCOME

The family will cope effectively with their loss and will adapt positively to their infant's special needs

Outcome measurement criteria

☐ Demonstration of progress through the stages of grief

☐ Absence of assigned guilt or blame among family members

☐ Demonstration of emotional support among family members

☐ Verbalization of an accurate understanding of the infant's condition

☐ Verbalization of an understanding of the infant's prognosis and treatment plan

☐ Involvement in the infant's care

☐ Demonstration of safe care of the infant

☐ Demonstration of attachment behaviors

Key interventions

• Establish a supportive, caring environment when the family initially is informed of the infant's condition. Allow time for family members to express initial concerns. Encourage them to ask questions; answer briefly and factually in the initial stages.

• Facilitate early family viewing and visits with the infant.

• Help the family explore the infant. Point out positive aspects of the infant's body and well-being.

- When feasible, touch the infant gently and lovingly to demonstrate acceptance of the infant for family members who may be experiencing shock, fear, and withdrawal.

- Teach the family how to touch the infant, if necessary.

- Provide an accepting environment for the family to express their feelings and fears. Help them recognize that part of their response is normal grief. Assist them in feeling comfortable with their shock, anger, disbelief, denial, depression, or withdrawal.

- Encourage family members to share their feelings and concerns with each other and health care team members frequently. Remind them not to become victims of persistent feelings of guilt or blame.

- Encourage family members to be compassionate and supportive with each other. Reinforce that each individual's adaptation is unique.

- When the family is ready for further knowledge about their infant's treatment and prognosis, help them obtain accurate information. Answer their questions and address their concerns.

- Use pictures to help the family visualize the effects of surgical correction of spina bifida.

- Encourage family members to take an active role in the infant's care. Facilitate visits with the infant whenever they desire.

- Teach family members how to feed the infant safely. Demonstrate the use of appropriate feeding techniques and equipment.

- Explain the importance of maintaining the skin integrity over bony prominences and the sac. Teach family members to massage areas of potential breakdown. Instruct them to notify the health care professional if skin breakdown occurs.

- Observe for persistent signs of lack of attachment, such as emotional withdrawal from the infant, resistance to infant care, distortion of the prognosis, or fear of taking the infant home.

- Refer the family with attachment difficulties to community agencies as needed.

- Refer the family to a support group for parents of infants with congenital defects. Facilitate the family's participation in the support group.

Substance withdrawal

Infant's physiologic recovery from the mother's antepartal use of substances, including drugs and alcohol. Such use of alcohol can lead to fetal alcohol syndrome, which can cause microcephaly, intrauterine growth retardation (IUGR), short palpebral fissures, and varying degrees of mental retardation.

NURSING DIAGNOSIS

Altered protection related to the physiologic effects of substance withdrawal

DESIRED PATIENT OUTCOME

The infant will remain free from injury caused by substance withdrawal

Outcome measurement criteria

☐ Absence of seizures

☐ Absence of respiratory distress

☐ Reduction of irritability

☐ Stabilization of body temperature

☐ Adequate nutritional intake

Key interventions

• Assess for factors that increase the infant's risk of substance withdrawal, such as maternal report of drug or alcohol use, signs of maternal drug or alcohol use, maternal malnutrition, maternal infection, history of maternal sexually transmitted disease, poor prenatal care, preterm labor and delivery, low Apgar scores, and infant resuscitation at delivery.

- Observe for characteristic signs of fetal alcohol syndrome, such as small-for-gestational-age status, IUGR, short palpebral fissures, a vertical ridge in the upper lip, a hypoplastic maxilla, and abnormal palmar creases.

- Observe the infant for signs of respiratory distress, including tachypnea, shallow respirations, nasal flaring, sternal retractions, excessive respiratory secretions, and periods of apnea.

- Observe for central nervous system signs of withdrawal, such as hypertonicity, hyperactivity, hyperirritability, increased reflexes, excessive sneezing, restless sleep, tremors, twitching, uncoordinated mouth and tongue movements, muscular rigidity, arching of the back, and seizures.

- Decrease physiologic stressors by providing a thermally neutral environment, providing nonnutritive sucking, and minimizing physical stimulation.

- Notify the health care professional of signs of suspected drug or alcohol withdrawal in the infant.

- Administer medications as prescribed to reduce hyperactivity, control seizures, and manage respiratory distress.

- Administer oxygen as prescribed to the infant with respiratory distress.

- Gently suction excessive respiratory secretions from the infant's oropharynx and nasopharynx.

- Place the infant in a side-lying position and elevate the head of the crib slightly to promote ease of breathing and secretion drainage.

NURSING DIAGNOSIS

High risk for altered nutrition: less than body requirements, related to uncoordinated sucking and swallowing, vomiting, and diarrhea

DESIRED PATIENT OUTCOME

The infant will obtain sufficient nutrients to support growth and development

Outcome measurement criteria

☐ Intake of 110 to 150 calories/kg/day

☐ Fluid intake of 140 to 160 ml/kg/day

☐ Little or no vomiting or diarrhea

☐ Urine specific gravity of 1.001 to 1.020

☐ Absence of signs of dehydration

☐ Weight gain of 0.4 to 0.5 oz (10 to 15 g) per day in a preterm infant; 0.7 to 1.1 oz (20 to 30 g) per day in a full-term infant

Key interventions

• Administer I.V. fluids as prescribed to support the infant through the acute phase of substance withdrawal.

• Document fluid intake and urine output, weighing diapers to accurately assess urine output.

• Assess the infant's ability to coordinate sucking and swallowing.

• Calculate the infant's caloric and fluid requirements based on daily weight.

• Offer frequent, small feedings of 5 to 10 ml if the infant displays signs of GI irritability. Use a soft nipple with a large hole. Provide feedings in a darkened, quiet environment with the infant well-swaddled to decrease environmental stimulation. Document the infant's response to each feeding.

• Estimate the quantity of any emesis and residual gastric contents. For the infant with vomiting and diarrhea, provide half-strength feedings as prescribed.

- Place the infant in a side-lying position with the head of the crib elevated slightly after feedings to decrease the risk of vomiting and aspiration.

- Measure and document urine specific gravity. Notify the health care professional of increasing specific gravity.

- Assess for signs of dehydration, such as decreased skin turgor, depressed fontanels, and weight loss.

- Weigh the infant at the same time every day, using the same scale. Document weight changes so that the infant's progress can be tracked easily.

- Provide nonnutritive sucking time for the infant to promote coordination of sucking and swallowing and to provide comfort.

NURSING DIAGNOSIS

High risk for impaired skin integrity related to hyperactivity and diarrhea

DESIRED PATIENT OUTCOME

The infant will display uninterrupted skin integrity

Outcome measurement criteria

- ☐ Little or no excoriation on the face or bony prominences
- ☐ Dry, clean perianal area
- ☐ Absence of signs of infection in abraded or excoriated areas

Key interventions

- Use soft bedding or sheepskin under the infant, especially under the face.
- Keep all bedding clean and dry.

- Change soiled diapers frequently to avoid perianal irritation. Use diapers that readily absorb liquid and apply them loosely to improve air circulation to tender skin. Occasionally, leave the perianal area open to the air to promote drying.

- Treat excoriated areas with ointment or occlusive transparent dressing as prescribed.

- Place mittens over the infant's hands to prevent skin damage from fingernails.

- Position the infant to avoid pressure on damaged skin surfaces.

- Observe damaged skin for increasing redness, edema, and drainage, which may signal infection. Notify the health care professional if such signs occur.

- Promote rest and decrease hyperactivity by swaddling the infant, decreasing environmental stimulation, providing for nonnutritive sucking, and administering medications as prescribed.

NURSING DIAGNOSIS

High risk for altered parenting related to the infant's difficulty in being consoled, parental lack of information about effective parenting techniques, and maternal history of substance abuse

DESIRED PATIENT OUTCOME

The parents will care for the infant effectively and knowledgeably

Outcome measurement criteria

☐ Verbalization of an understanding of the infant's difficulty in being consoled

☐ Demonstration of techniques for comforting the infant

☐ Verbalization of an understanding of the infant's need for rest periods

☐ Demonstration of effective techniques for infant feeding, bathing, and dressing

☐ Use of external resources for assistance with infant care and substance dependence

Key interventions

• Establish a rapport with the infant's parents. Encourage them to discuss their feelings, ask questions, and identify concerns.

• Teach the parents about the infant's behaviors related to substance withdrawal, such as hyperactivity, hyperirritability, and difficulty in being consoled. Explain that these behaviors may be short-term or long-term.

• Help the parents recognize signs of infant overstimulation, such as yawning, excessive high-pitched crying, and restlessness.

• Encourage the parents to try different methods of consolation. Explain that, at times, the infant may be comforted by being caressed, rocked, cuddled, and talked to and that, at other times, the infant may be comforted by being swaddled and placed in an environment with little external stimuli. Explain how nonnutritive sucking can comfort the infant.

• Model nurturing behaviors, such as cuddling, swaddling, and caressing, and teach the parents how to perform them, as needed.

• Inform the parents about the infant's nutritional needs and feeding habits. Show them how to feed the infant appropriately.

• Teach the parents how to provide routine infant care. Encourage them to participate in the hospitalized infant's care and evaluate their interaction with the infant.

- Observe for persistent signs of lack of attachment, such as emotional withdrawal from the infant, resistance to infant care, distortion of the prognosis, or fear of taking the infant home.

- Encourage the infant's mother to discuss her plans for managing drug or alcohol dependence.

- Refer the parents to support services for management of drug or alcohol dependence, parenting classes, home health agencies, and adoption or foster care services as needed.

- Make referrals to child protective services as needed.

Talipes deformity

Congenital deformity that causes the affected foot to be twisted out of its normal position or shape.

NURSING DIAGNOSIS

High risk for impaired tissue integrity related to foot casts

DESIRED PATIENT OUTCOME

The infant will exhibit intact tissue around and under the casts

Outcome measurement criteria

- ☐ Vital signs within normal limits
- ☐ Capillary refill time of less than 4 seconds in toes and feet
- ☐ Warm feet with positive peripheral pulses
- ☐ Absence of edema
- ☐ Absence of abrasions at cast edges

Key interventions

- Reposition the infant at least every 2 hours while the casts dry. Leave the casts uncovered and use a fan to speed drying if the infant is sufficiently warm.
- Elevate the legs on pillows while the casts dry. Monitor the infant's respirations carefully while in this position.
- Frequently monitor and document the infant's vital signs, capillary refill time, skin color and temperature, and peripheral pulses. Also check for edema in the affected areas.

- Inspect the skin distal to the cast edges, particularly noting signs of breakdown.
- Report any abnormal assessment findings.

NURSING DIAGNOSIS

Ineffective family coping: compromised, related to the loss of the idealized infant and lack of knowledge about caring for an infant with corrective casts

DESIRED PATIENT OUTCOME

The family will cope effectively with feelings about their infant's condition and will provide appropriate care

Outcome measurement criteria

- ☐ Expression of feelings about the infant's condition
- ☐ Demonstration of mutual support among family members
- ☐ Verbalization of an accurate understanding of talipes deformity
- ☐ Demonstration of appropriate physical care and social stimulation for the infant
- ☐ Demonstration of attachment behaviors

Key interventions

- Establish a supportive relationship with the family. Encourage them to express their feelings about the infant's condition.
- Provide support to family members who may be grieving over the loss of the idealized infant. Point out positive aspects of the infant's body and well-being.
- Reassure the family that early recognition and treatment of talipes deformity increases ultimate success.

- Help the family obtain accurate information about their infant's particular talipes deformity and its treatment. Provide written and verbal information as needed.

- Emphasize the importance of casts as the initial intervention.

- Teach family members to assess the infant's feet and legs for signs of problems with the casts. Instruct them to assess the area around the casts daily for signs of irritation or skin breakdown. Show them how to reduce skin irritation, if needed, by lightly padding the cast edges.

- Teach family members not to apply powders or lotions under the cast edges. Show them how to care for the cast edges to prevent contamination and irritation, for example, by altering of the cast edges with adhesive bandages or strips of tape or disposable diapers.

- Explain the infant's need for auditory, visual, and tactile stimulation. Encourage the family to provide appropriate stimulation.

- Demonstrate safe methods of physical interaction with the infant.

- Observe for persistent signs of lack of attachment, such as emotional withdrawal from the infant, resistance to infant care, distortion of the prognosis, or fear of taking the infant home.

- Refer the family with attachment difficulties to community agencies as needed.

Tracheoesophageal fistula and esophageal atresia

Congenital defect in which an abnormal opening exists between the trachea and esophagus, an abnormal closure of the esophagus creates a blind esophageal pouch, or both.

NURSING DIAGNOSIS

Ineffective airway clearance related to congenital defects that interfere with the infant's ability to swallow secretions

DESIRED PATIENT OUTCOME

The infant will maintain a patent airway

Outcome measurement criteria

☐ Respiratory rate of 30 to 60 breaths/minute

☐ Absence of signs of respiratory distress

☐ Normal breath sounds on auscultation

☐ Absence of cyanosis

☐ Pulse oximetry values of more than 95%

☐ Arterial blood gas (ABG) levels within normal limits

Key interventions

• Be alert for signs of tracheoesophageal fistula or esophageal atresia, such as excessive production of bubbling mucus secretions, continuous drooling, choking on secretions, abdominal distention beginning shortly after delivery, respiratory distress, or immediate regurgitation of initial feeding.

- Perform oropharyngeal, nasopharyngeal, and endotracheal suction as needed to prevent secretion accumulation in the airway.

- Adjust a nasogastric tube to low intermittent suction to maintain decompression of the blind pouch.

- Administer nothing by mouth (NPO), as ordered.

- Keep resuscitation equipment at the bedside.

- Place the infant in a thermally neutral environment to decrease the metabolic demand.

- Elevate the infant's head 20 to 40 degrees to decrease gastric reflux into the trachea. Place the infant in a prone or side-lying position, if tolerated, to decrease the risk of aspiration and promote decompression of the abdomen.

- Anticipate the infant's needs to prevent crying, which can increase air ingestion into the blind pouch and lead to increased respiratory distress.

- Avoid the use of a pacifier because it can increase the production of oral secretions.

- Assess the respiratory rate, depth, and effort. Auscultate the lungs to detect adventitious breath sounds. Document findings and notify the health care professional of signs of respiratory distress, such as increasing tachypnea, nasal flaring, grunting, accessory muscle use, decreased breath sounds, or crackles.

- Observe for increasing cyanosis, and monitor pulse oximetry values. Document findings and report signs of deterioration.

- Review ABG levels as ordered, particularly noting hypoxia, hypercapnia, or acidosis.

- Administer oxygen as ordered. Assist with intubation and mechanical ventilation as needed.

- Administer antibiotics as prescribed to prevent or correct pneumonitis.

NURSING DIAGNOSIS

High risk for altered nutrition: less than body requirements, related to NPO status required by tracheoesophageal fistula and esophageal atresia

DESIRED PATIENT OUTCOME

The infant will obtain sufficient nutrients to support growth

Outcome measurement criteria

☐ Weight gain of 0.5 to 1.1 oz (15 to 30 g) per day

☐ Intake of 110 to 150 calories/kg/day

☐ Serum glucose level of 45 to 90 mg/dl

Key interventions

- Weigh the infant at the same time every day, using the same scale. Document weight changes so that the infant's progress can be tracked easily.

- Calculate caloric and fluid needs every day based on the infant's current weight.

- Monitor the infant's blood glucose level to determine if sufficient energy is available to meet metabolic demands.

- Administer I.V. fluids that contain glucose and provide total parenteral nutrition as prescribed.

- Maintain the infant's NPO status as ordered until corrective surgery has been performed.

- Notify the health care professional of loss of more than 2% of body weight in 24 hours.

NURSING DIAGNOSIS

High risk for fluid volume deficit related to NPO status and frequent suctioning

DESIRED PATIENT OUTCOME
The infant will display adequate fluid volume

Outcome measurement criteria
☐ Urine output of at least 2 ml/kg/hour

☐ Urine specific gravity of 1.001 to 1.020

☐ Absence of signs of dehydration

☐ Fluid intake that approximates output

Key interventions
- Maintain a thermally neutral environment to decrease insensible fluid loss.

- Monitor and record the infant's fluid intake and urine output hourly. Weigh diapers to measure urine output accurately. Document intake and output and calculate the need for fluid replacement based on this information.

- Assess the infant's urine specific gravity. Note increasing specific gravity, which may indicate dehydration.

- Assess for other signs of dehydration, including depressed fontanels, lethargy, decreased skin turgor, and dry mucous membranes.

- Notify the health care professional of the infant's fluid volume status as ordered.

- Administer I.V. fluids as prescribed.

NURSING DIAGNOSIS
Anxiety (parental) related to the unknown outcome of surgery

DESIRED PATIENT OUTCOME
The parents will display reduced anxiety

Outcome measurement criteria

☐ Expression of concerns about the infant's condition

☐ Verbalization of an understanding of tracheoesophageal fistula and esophageal atresia and their treatment

☐ Demonstration of appropriate infant care

☐ Demonstration of attachment behaviors

Key interventions

• Establish a supportive relationship with the parents. Encourage them to express their concerns, fears, and other feelings.

• Assess the parents' knowledge of their infant's congenital defect. Help them obtain accurate information about its treatment and prognosis. Encourage the parents to ask questions.

• Update the parents about the infant's condition and progress.

• Teach the parents, if needed, how to touch and caress the infant. Model acceptance of the infant for the parents.

• Demonstrate how to care for the infant. Then have the parents return the demonstration.

• Explain the significance of any monitoring equipment used.

• Observe for persistent signs of lack of attachment, such as emotional withdrawal from the infant, resistance to infant care, distortion of the prognosis, or fear of taking the infant home.

• Refer the parents with attachment difficulties to community agencies as needed.

APPENDIX 1

NANDA taxonomy of nursing diagnoses

The currently accepted classification system for nursing diagnoses is that of the North American Nursing Diagnosis Association (NANDA), as shown in *NANDA Nursing Diagnoses: Definitions and Classification 1992-1993*. It is organized around nine human response patterns: exchanging, communicating, relating, valuing, choosing, moving, perceiving, knowing, and feeling.

The complete taxonomic structure is listed here. The series of numbers before each diagnosis is its classification number, used to determine the placement of the diagnosis within the taxonomy. The number of digits delineates the level of abstraction of the nursing diagnosis (more specific diagnoses are assigned longer numbers).

Pattern 1. Exchanging

1.1.2.1	Altered nutrition: More than body requirements
1.1.2.2	Altered nutrition: Less than body requirements
1.1.2.3	Altered nutrition: Potential for more than body requirements
1.2.1.1	High risk for infection
1.2.2.1	High risk for altered body temperature
1.2.2.2	Hypothermia
1.2.2.3	Hyperthermia
1.2.2.4	Ineffective thermoregulation
1.2.3.1	Dysreflexia
1.3.1.1	Constipation
1.3.1.1.1	Perceived constipation
1.3.1.1.2	Colonic constipation
1.3.1.2	Diarrhea
1.3.1.3	Bowel incontinence
1.3.2	Altered urinary elimination
1.3.2.1.1	Stress incontinence
1.3.2.1.2	Reflex incontinence
1.3.2.1.3	Urge incontinence
1.3.2.1.4	Functional incontinence
1.3.2.1.5	Total incontinence
1.3.2.2	Urinary retention
1.4.1.1	Altered (specify type) tissue perfusion (renal, cerebral, cardiopulmonary, gastrointestinal, peripheral)
1.4.1.2.1	Fluid volume excess
1.4.1.2.2.1	Fluid volume deficit
1.4.1.2.2.2	High risk for fluid volume deficit
1.4.2.1	Decreased cardiac output
1.5.1.1	Impaired gas exchange
1.5.1.2	Ineffective airway clearance
1.5.1.3	Ineffective breathing pattern
1.5.1.3.1	Inability to sustain spontaneous ventilation
1.5.1.3.2	Dysfunctional ventilatory weaning response
1.6.1	High risk for injury
1.6.1.1	High risk for suffocation
1.6.1.2	High risk for poisoning
1.6.1.3	High risk for trauma
1.6.1.4	High risk for aspiration
1.6.1.5	High risk for disuse syndrome
1.6.2	Altered protection
1.6.2.1	Impaired tissue integrity
1.6.2.1.1	Altered oral mucous membrane
1.6.2.1.2.1	Impaired skin integrity
1.6.2.1.2.2	High risk for impaired skin integrity

Pattern 2. Communicating

2.1.1.1	Impaired verbal communication

Pattern 3. Relating

3.1.1	Impaired social interaction
3.1.2	Social isolation
3.2.1	Altered role performance
3.2.1.1.1	Altered parenting
3.2.1.1.2	High risk for altered parenting
3.2.1.2.1	Sexual dysfunction
3.2.2	Altered family processes
3.2.2.1	Caregiver role strain

3.2.2.2	High risk for caregiver role strain	6.5.4	Toileting self-care deficit
3.2.3.1	Parental role conflict	6.6	Altered growth and development
3.3	Altered sexuality patterns	6.7	Relocation stress syndrome

Pattern 4. Valuing

4.1.1	Spiritual distress (distress of the human spirit)

Pattern 5. Choosing

5.1.1.1	Ineffective individual coping
5.1.1.1.1	Impaired adjustment
5.1.1.1.2	Defensive coping
5.1.1.1.3	Ineffective denial
5.1.2.1.1	Ineffective family coping: Disabling
5.1.2.1.2	Ineffective family coping: Compromised
5.1.2.2	Family coping: Potential for growth
5.2.1	Ineffective management of therapeutic regimen (individual)
5.2.1.1	Noncompliance (specify)
5.3.1.1	Decisional conflict (specify)
5.4	Health-seeking behaviors (specify)

Pattern 6. Moving

6.1.1.1	Impaired physical mobility
6.1.1.1.1	High risk for peripheral neurovascular dysfunction
6.1.1.2	Activity intolerance
6.1.1.2.1	Fatigue
6.1.1.3	High risk for activity intolerance
6.2.1	Sleep pattern disturbance
6.3.1.1	Diversional activity deficit
6.4.1.1	Impaired home maintenance management
6.4.2	Altered health maintenance
6.5.1	Feeding self-care deficit
6.5.1.1	Impaired swallowing
6.5.1.2	Ineffective breast-feeding
6.5.1.2.1	Interrupted breast-feeding
6.5.1.3	Effective breast-feeding
6.5.1.4	Ineffective infant feeding pattern
6.5.2	Bathing or hygiene self-care deficit
6.5.3	Dressing or grooming self-care deficit

Pattern 7. Perceiving

7.1.1	Body image disturbance
7.1.2	Self-esteem disturbance
7.1.2.1	Chronic low self-esteem
7.1.2.2	Situational low self-esteem
7.1.3	Personal identity disturbance
7.2	Sensory or perceptual alterations (specify visual, auditory, kinesthetic, gustatory, tactile, olfactory)
7.2.1.1	Unilateral neglect
7.3.1	Hopelessness
7.3.2	Powerlessness

Pattern 8. Knowing

8.1.1	Knowledge deficit (specify)
8.3	Altered thought processes

Pattern 9. Feeling

9.1.1	Pain
9.1.1.1	Chronic pain
9.2.1.1	Dysfunctional grieving
9.2.1.2	Anticipatory grieving
9.2.2	High risk for violence: Self-directed or directed at others
9.2.2.1	High risk for self-mutilation
9.2.3	Post-trauma response
9.2.3.1	Rape-trauma syndrome
9.2.3.1.1	Rape-trauma syndrome: Compound reaction
9.2.3.1.2	Rape-trauma syndrome: Silent reaction
9.3.1	Anxiety
9.3.2	Fear

© North American Nursing Diagnosis Association (1992). *NANDA Nursing Diagnoses: Definitions and Classification 1992-1993*. Philadelphia: NANDA.

APPENDIX 2

Common nursing diagnoses in maternal-infant care

The following list summarizes the nursing diagnoses that appear in this book, which are among the most common diagnoses in maternal-infant nursing.

ANTEPARTAL PERIOD

Adolescent pregnancy

- Anxiety related to parenthood, the effect of parenthood on relationships, and labor and delivery
- Altered family processes related to the stress of adolescent pregnancy
- Ineffective management of therapeutic regimen related to inadequate knowledge of prenatal care and inconsistent participation in it
- High risk for altered parenting related to inadequate support systems, lack of knowledge, and unrealistic expectations

Advanced maternal age during pregnancy

- Altered family processes related to integration of the expected infant into established patterns of family functioning
- Health-seeking behaviors (appropriate self-care) related to involvement in the therapeutic regimen during pregnancy

Anemia

- Altered nutrition: less than body requirements, related to inadequate iron intake and increased need for iron

Cervical incompetence

- Anxiety related to unknown pregnancy outcome secondary to cervical incompetence

Diabetes mellitus

- Fear related to the effect of diabetes on maternal and fetal well-being
- Ineffective management of therapeutic regimen related to lack of knowledge about and complexity of the regimen
- High risk for injury related to unstable blood glucose level

Discomforts of the first trimester

- Altered nutrition: less than body requirements, related to nausea and vomiting in early pregnancy
- Altered urinary elimination pattern related to urinary frequency and urgency caused by the physiological changes that occur during early pregnancy
- High risk for infection related to the physiological effects of pregnancy on the urinary tract
- Fatigue related to the increased physiologic demands of early pregnancy

- Altered sexuality patterns related to pregnancy discomforts and fear about the effects of sexual activity on the fetus
- Pain related to headaches caused by the physiological effects of early pregnancy
- High risk for injury related to frequent dizziness and fainting caused by the effects of early pregnancy

Discomforts of the second trimester
- Pain related to heartburn, varicosities, or hemorrhoids caused by the physiologic changes of pregnancy
- Constipation related to the physiologic changes of pregnancy and painful hemorrhoids
- High risk for injury (fetal or maternal) related to the effects of supine hypotension

Discomforts of the third trimester
- Pain related to round ligament stetching, leg cramps, perineal pressure, Braxton Hicks contractions, and backache secondary to advanced pregnancy
- Activity intolerance related to dyspnea secondary to the physiologic effects of advanced pregnancy
- Sleep pattern disturbance related to insomnia secondary to advanced pregnancy
- Altered peripheral tissue perfusion related to edema caused by the physiologic effects of pregnancy

Ectopic pregnancy
- Pain related to the effects of tubal rupture from ectopic pregnancy or surgery for it
- Fluid volume deficit related to excessive fluid loss secondary to complications of ectopic pregnancy or surgery for it
- High risk for dysfunctional grieving related to the effects of pregnancy loss or salpingectomy

Elective termination of pregnancy
- Decisional conflict related to ambivalence about pregnancy termination
- Fear related to pregnancy-termination surgery and its implications for future pregnancies
- High risk for infection related to postoperative complications of elective termination of pregnancy

Human immunodeficiency virus infection
- Ineffective individual coping related to difficulty accepting human immunodeficiency virus (HIV)-positive status
- Ineffective management of treatment regimen related to lack of knowledge and skill to manage HIV infection, medication regimen, and infection control
- High risk for infection related to decreased resistance secondary to immune system compromise by HIV infection
- Hopelessness related to the terminal nature of HIV infection

- High risk for infection (fetal) related to HIV exposure from the mother

Hyperemesis gravidarum
- Altered nutrition: less than body requirements, related to abnormal fluid loss caused by hyperemesis gravidarum
- Activity intolerance related to inadequate nutrition and fluid and electrolyte imbalance
- Fear related to the effects of hyperemesis gravidarum on maternal and fetal well-being

Multifetal pregnancy
- Ineffective individual and family coping related to the increased physiologic and therapeutic demands imposed by multifetal pregnancy
- Parental role conflict related to uncertainty about the ability to care for more than one infant

Placenta previa
- Fear related to the effects of placenta previa on the pregnancy
- Diversional activity deficit related to imposed bed rest secondary to placenta previa
- Altered peripheral tissue perfusion related to excessive blood loss caused by placenta previa

Pregnancy-induced hypertension
- Ineffective management of therapeutic regimen related to lack of knowledge about pregnancy-induced hypertension (PIH) and the complexity of its treatment
- Diversional activity deficit related to imposed bed rest secondary to PIH
- High risk for injury (maternal and fetal) related to the effects of preeclampsia or its treatment

Premature rupture of membranes
- High risk for infection related to premature rupture of membranes (PROM)
- Altered family processes related to situational crisis secondary to PROM
- Fear related to unknown pregnancy outcome

Preterm labor
- Fear related to the unknown effects of preterm labor on the pregnancy outcome
- Ineffective management of therapeutic regimen related to lack of knowledge about and complexity of therapy for preterm labor
- Diversional activity deficit related to imposed bed rest secondary to preterm labor
- Constipation related to decreased GI activity caused by imposed bed rest and the adverse effects of tocolytics

Sexually transmitted diseases
- Ineffective management of therapeutic regimen related to lack of knowledge about disease transmission, treatment, and prevention

- Personal identity disturbance related to the impact of a sexually transmitted disease (STD)

- Altered family processes related to the effects of the STD on family relationships

Spontaneous abortion
- High risk for dysfunctional grieving related to pregnancy loss

- High risk for fluid volume deficit related to excessive blood loss secondary to spontaneous abortion

Substance abuse during pregnancy
- High risk for ineffective management of therapeutic regimen related to addiction or dependence, inconsistent participation in prenatal care, and lack of knowledge of the potentially harmful effects of substance abuse

- High risk for ineffective individual coping related to inability to manage stress without the use of drugs

TORCH infections
- Anticipatory grieving related to the infection's potential effects on the fetus

- Ineffective management of therapeutic regimen related to inadequate knowledge of the cause, treatment, prevention, and risks associated with the infection

- High risk for infection (fetal) related to exposure to organisms from the pregnant patient

Trauma or battering during pregnancy
- Pain related to injuries secondary to trauma or battering

- Fear related to the actual or perceived fetal effects of the maternal physical injury

- High risk for injury (fetal) related to preterm labor or abruptio placentae secondary to physical injuries from or surgical intervention for trauma or battering

- Hopelessness related to prolonged exposure to violence

Urinary tract infection
- Pain related to urinary tract infection (UTI)

- Ineffective management of therapeutic regimen related to insufficient knowledge of the cause, prevention, treatment, and risks of UTI

Vaginitis
- Impaired tissue integrity related to pruritus, excoriation, and inflammation caused by vaginitis

- Altered sexuality patterns related to dyspareunia from vaginitis

INTRAPARTAL PERIOD

Abruptio placentae
- Pain related to increased intrauterine pressure secondary to bleeding from abruptio placentae

- Altered fetal tissue perfusion related to decreased placental circulation secondary to abruptio placentae

- High risk for fluid volume deficit related to excessive blood loss secondary to concealed or frank hemorrhage

- Fear related to inadequate knowledge about treatment for abruptio placentae and the disorder's potential effects on maternal and fetal well-being

Amniotic fluid embolism

- Inability to sustain spontaneous ventilation related to compromised cardiopulmonary status secondary to amniotic fluid embolism

- Altered placental and peripheral tissue perfusion related to compromised cardiovascular status secondary to amniotic fluid embolism

- Fear related to inadequate knowledge about treatment and the potential effects of amniotic fluid embolism on maternal and fetal well-being

- High risk for fluid volume deficit related to excessive blood loss secondary to altered clotting mechanism

- High risk for infection related to the use of invasive monitoring devices

Cesarean delivery

- Fear related to perceived threat to self and lack of knowledge about cesarean delivery

- Situational low self-esteem related to failure to accomplish vaginal delivery

Dystocia

- Pain related to intense uterine contractions or prolonged labor

- Ineffective individual coping related to ineffective breathing patterns, fatigue, fear, or lack of adequate support during labor and delivery

- Situational low self-esteem related to inability to complete labor and delivery as planned

- High risk for fluid volume deficit related to restricted oral intake, vomiting, and increased insensible fluid loss during prolonged labor

- High risk for infection related to invasive monitoring and frequent assessment

- High risk for injury (maternal) related to soft tissue damage secondary to difficult labor and delivery

- High risk for injury (fetal) related to prolonged compression against maternal pelvic structures, decreased uteroplacental circulation, or shoulder dystocia

Eclampsia

- High risk for injury (maternal and fetal) related to the effects of seizures

- Altered fetal tissue perfusion related to a rapid decrease in available oxygen secondary to maternal seizures

- High risk for aspiration related to seizures

- High risk for fluid volume deficit related to excessive blood loss secondary to complications of eclampsia
- High risk for infection related to use of invasive monitoring and vaginal examinations
- Fear related to lack of knowledge about eclampsia's treatment and the potential effects on maternal and fetal well-being

Electronic fetal monitoring
- Anxiety related to lack of knowledge about electronic fetal monitoring
- Pain related to the perceived need to remain immobile and the presence of monitor attachments
- High risk for injury (fetal) related to hypoxia secondary to persistent nonreassuring FHR patterns or the absence of uterine resting tone

HELLP syndrome
- High risk for injury (maternal and fetal) related to abnormal cardiovascular function and multisystem organ dysfunction secondary to HELLP syndrome
- Fear related to lack of knowledge about treatment for HELLP syndrome and the disorder's potential effects on maternal and fetal well-being
- High risk for dysfunctional grieving related to maternal and fetal morbidity and possible mortality secondary to HELLP syndrome
- Altered family processes related to the effects of a critical maternal and fetal illness
- High risk for infection related to the use of an invasive monitoring device

Induction of labor
- Anxiety related to lack of knowledge about labor induction
- High risk for situational low self-esteem related to feelings of failure secondary to the need for labor induction
- High risk for altered placental tissue perfusion related to uterine hyperstimulation caused by labor induction

Infections
- High risk for infection (fetal) related to HIV exposure from the mother
- High risk for infection (fetal) related to exposure to organisms that cause TORCH infections from the pregnant patient

Labor and vaginal delivery, common course
- Fear related to unfamiliarity with labor
- Pain related to increasing intensity and duration of uterine contractions
- High risk for fluid volume deficit related to restricted oral intake, increased fluid loss during labor, and inadequate fluid intake
- High risk for injury (maternal and fetal) related to complications of analgesia or anesthesia

- Ineffective individual coping related to ineffective breathing patterns, fatigue, fear, or lack of a support person

- High risk for low self-esteem related to loss of control of emotions and elimination

- High risk for fluid volume deficit related to abnormal bleeding secondary to uterine changes during the fourth stage of labor

- Altered family processes related to the addition of a new family member

Manual extraction of the placenta

- Pain related to the effects of manipulations used in manual extraction of the placenta

- High risk for fluid volume deficit related to abnormal uterine bleeding caused by manual extraction of the placenta

- High risk for infection related to intrauterine exposure to pathogens during manual extraction of the placenta

Postdatism

- High risk for injury (fetal) related to hypoxia secondary to decreased uteroplacental function

Precipitous labor and delivery

- High risk for injury (maternal and fetal) related to the extreme force and increased frequency of uterine contractions secondary to precipitous labor

- High risk for altered fetal tissue perfusion related to inadequate uterine resting tone during precipitous labor

- High risk for infection related to lacerations of cervical, vaginal, perianal, or periurethral tissue during precipitous labor and delivery

- Ineffective individual and family coping related to a panic reaction to precipitous labor and delivery

Umbilical cord prolapse

- High risk for altered fetal tissue perfusion related to blood flow occlusion secondary to prolapsed umbilical cord

- Fear related to lack of knowledge about treatment for umbilical cord prolapse and its potential effects on fetal well-being

Uterine rupture

- Altered fetal tissue perfusion related to decreased placental circulation secondary to uterine rupture

- High risk for fluid volume deficit related to excessive blood loss secondary to concealed or apparent hemorrhage from uterine rupture

- High risk for infection related to altered skin integrity and blood loss secondary to uterine rupture and cesarean delivery

Vaginal birth after cesarean

- Fear related to labor and the potential for repeat cesarean delivery

POSTPARTAL PERIOD

Bottle-feeding

- High risk for anxiety (maternal) related to inexperience with bottle-feeding

- High risk for ineffective infant feeding pattern related to inadequate knowledge of bottle-feeding techniques and practices

- High risk for altered nutrition: less or more than body requirements, related to inadequate parental knowledge of the infant's nutritional needs

Breast-feeding

- High risk for anxiety (maternal) related to inexperience with breast-feeding

- High risk for ineffective breast-feeding related to inadequate knowledge of the benefits of breast-feeding

- High risk for ineffective breast-feeding related to inadequate knowledge of feeding techniques and practices

- High risk for interrupted breast-feeding related to cracked, sore, or inverted nipples, breast engorgement, mastitis, lack of social support, or separation from the infant

- High risk for situational low self-esteem related to inadequate milk production

- High risk for altered sexuality patterns related to ambivalence of the sexual partners secondary to lactation

Family adaptation to an ill infant

- Grieving related to the loss of the idealized infant

- Altered parenting related to the demands of caring for an ill infant

Family adaptation to a well infant

- Family coping: potential for growth, related to the perceived need to learn infant care

- Altered family processes related to infant care demands

- Family coping: potential for growth, related to the perceived need to promote sibling adaptation

Family adaptation to loss of an infant

- High risk for dysfunctional grieving related to the death of an infant

- High risk for ineffective family coping: disabling, related to the inability to resolve grief over the infant's death

Mastitis

- High risk for interrupted breast-feeding related to pain, dissatisfaction with breast-feeding, and situational low self-esteem

- High risk for ineffective management of therapeutic regimen related to inadequate knowledge about the medication regimen, self-care, and infant-feeding practices during mastitis

Postpartal common course

- High risk for injury related to the effects of fluid loss

- High risk for infection related to interruption of the first line of defense secondary to delivery
- Pain related to tissue trauma and the normal physiologic changes during the postpartal period
- Sleep pattern disturbance related to fatigue, facility routine, and infant care demands
- High risk for situational low self-esteem related to the discrepancy between the imagined and actual delivery, altered body image, and inexperience with infant care
- Altered urinary elimination related to the effects of birth trauma on the urinary tract and to postpartal diuresis
- High risk for constipation related to tissue trauma, hemorrhoids, and the normal physiologic changes during the postpartal period
- High risk for altered parenting related to incisional pain from cesarean delivery and unmet expectations of labor and delivery
- Impaired gas exchange related to shallow breathing and weak cough secondary to pain from the surgical incision
- Ineffective individual coping related to depression-induced inability to identify and express needs

Postpartal hemorrhage
- Fluid volume deficit related to excessive blood loss secondary to postpartal hemorrhage
- High risk for infection related to excessive blood loss and measures used to control postpartal hemorrhage
- High risk for altered parenting related to delayed attachment secondary to postpartal hemorrhage-induced fatigue

Postpartal infections
- High risk for infection (postpartal) related to chorioamnionitis
- High risk for fluid volume deficit related to excessive uterine bleeding secondary to chorioamnionitis-induced uterine atony
- High risk for injury related to possible bacteremic shock secondary to a postpartal infection
- Pain related to effects of infection
- High risk for altered parenting related to delayed attachment secondary to malaise and forced separation from the infant

Pulmonary embolus
- High risk for inability to sustain spontaneous ventilation related to compromised cardiopulmonary status secondary to pulmonary embolus
- Fear related to lack of knowledge about the disorder's treatment and potential effects

Urinary bladder distention

- Altered urinary elimination related to urine stasis secondary to mechanical trauma of the urinary tract, the effects of anesthesia, altered voiding reflex, postpartal diuresis, or bladder atony

Venous thrombosis

- Altered peripheral tissue perfusion related to obstruction of venous circulation secondary to venous thrombosis

- High risk for injury related to abnormal bleeding secondary to anticoagulant therapy

- Pain related to the effects of venous thrombosis

INFANT

Caput succedaneum

- Anxiety (parental) related to lack of knowledge about caput succedaneum

Cardiovascular defect, congenital

- High risk for injury related to the physiologic effects of a congenital cardiovascular defect

- Altered cardiopulmonary tissue perfusion related to decreased circulating oxygen secondary to a congenital cardiovascular heart defect

- High risk for altered nutrition: less than body requirements, related to fatigue and dyspnea during feedings

- Activity intolerance related to inadequate circulating oxygen

- Ineffective family coping: compromised, related to grief over the loss of the idealized infant and guilt, fear, anxiety, and lack of knowledge about the infant's condition

Cephalhematoma

- Anxiety (parental) related to lack of knowledge about cephalhematoma

Circumcision

- High risk for injury related to the effects of circumcision

- Anxiety (parental) related to lack of knowledge about appropriate care for the newly circumcised infant

Cleft lip or palate

- High risk for altered nutrition: less than body requirements, related to inability to suck adequately

- High risk for aspiration related to an inability to clear secretions or milk from the cleft palate and nasal mucous membranes

- Ineffective family coping: compromised, related to grief over the loss of the idealized infant and guilt, fear, anxiety, and lack of knowledge about the infant's condition

Cold stress

- Ineffective thermoregulation related to the infant's immature thermoregulatory mechanisms

- High risk for injury related to hyperthermia secondary to correction of hypothermia

Gastrointestinal obstruction, congenital

- High risk for fluid volume deficit related to vomiting secondary to GI obstruction
- Impaired gas exchange related to GI distention that creates abnormal pressure in the lungs
- High risk for infection related to aspiration of vomitus
- Anxiety (parental) related to the unknown outcome of surgery

Hip dysplasia, congenital

- Altered growth and development related to the effects of undiagnosed or untreated congenital hip dysplasia
- Ineffective family coping: compromised, related to grief over the loss of the idealized child and to the need for an abduction device

Human immunodeficiency virus infection

- Altered protection related to the effects of the mother's human immunodeficiency virus (HIV) infection and the infant's immature immune system
- High risk for altered parenting related to the infant's potential illness and lack of information about effective parenting techniques

Hydrocephalus

- High risk for injury related to increased head weight and size
- Ineffective family coping: compromised, related to grief over the loss of the idealized infant and guilt, fear, anxiety, and lack of knowledge about hydrocephalus

Hyperbilirubinemia

- High risk for injury related to the effects of elevated serum bilirubin level
- Altered protection related to the effects of phototherapy
- High risk for fluid volume deficit related to abnormal fluid loss secondary to phototherapy
- Anxiety (parental) related to lack of knowledge about hyperbilirubinemia and its treatment
- Interrupted breast-feeding related to the need for phototherapy secondary to breast-milk jaundice

Hypocalcemia

- High risk for injury related to hypocalcemia
- Anxiety (parental) related to lack of knowledge about hypocalcemia and its treatment

Hypoglycemia

- High risk for injury related to hypoglycemia
- Anxiety (parental) related to lack of knowledge about hypoglycemia and its treatment

Isoimmune hemolytic anemia

- High risk for injury related to the effects of isoimmune hemolytic anemia

- Altered family processes related to lack of knowledge about isoimmune hemolytic anemia and interruption of parent-infant attachment

Meconium aspiration syndrome

- Impaired gas exchange related to meconium aspirate in the respiratory tract

- High risk for infection related to invasive monitors used during the treatment of meconium aspiration syndrome (MAS)

- Altered family processes related to lack of knowledge about MAS and interruption of parent-infant attachment

Necrotizing enterocolitis

- High risk for injury related to the progression of necrosis

- Fluid volume deficit related to nothing-by-mouth status, the need for bowel rest, and abnormal fluid loss through vomiting and diarrhea

- High risk for altered nutrition: less than body requirements, related to treatment of necrotizing enterocolitis (NEC)

- Altered family processes related to lack of knowledge about NEC and interruption of parent-infant attachment

Peripheral nervous system injury

- High risk for injury related to birth trauma

- Anxiety (parental) related to disappointment with the infant's appearance, uncertainty about the prognosis, and lack of knowledge about the infant's care

Respiratory distress syndrome

- Impaired gas exchange related to inadequate lung surfactant and decreased alveolar perfusion secondary to prematurity

- Activity intolerance related to inadequate pulmonary function secondary to prematurity

- High risk for altered nutrition: less than body requirements, related to treatment for respiratory distress syndrome (RDS)

- High risk for infection related to use of invasive monitors during treatment for RDS

- Altered family processes related to lack of knowledge about RDS and interruption of parent-infant attachment

Sepsis neonatorum

- Altered protection related to the presence of infectious organisms and the infant's immature immune system

- Impaired gas exchange related to the physiologic effects of sepsis neonatorum

- High risk for fluid volume deficit related to the physiologic effects of sepsis neonatorum

- Altered family processes related to lack of knowledge about sepsis neonatorum and interruption of parent-infant attachment

Skeletal injury
- Pain related to skeletal injury and tissue trauma

Soft tissue injury
- Anxiety (parental) related to lack of knowledge about soft tissue injury

Spina bifida
- High risk for infection related to altered skin integrity over the protruding sac or over bony prominences
- Ineffective thermoregulation related to an open lesion on the spinal column
- Ineffective family coping: compromised, related to grief over the loss of the idealized infant and guilt, fear, anxiety, and lack of knowledge about spina bifida

Substance withdrawal
- Altered protection related to the physiologic effects of substance withdrawal
- High risk for altered nutrition: less than body requirements, related to uncoordinated sucking and swallowing, vomiting, and diarrhea
- High risk for impaired skin integrity related to hyperactivity and diarrhea
- High risk for altered parenting related to the infant's difficulty in being consoled, parental lack of knowledge about effective parenting techniques, and maternal history of substance abuse

Talipes deformity
- High risk for impaired tissue integrity related to foot casts
- Ineffective family coping: compromised, related to the loss of the idealized infant and lack of knowledge about caring for an infant with corrective casts

Tracheoesophageal fistula and esophageal atresia
- Ineffective airway clearance related to congenital defects that interfere with the infant's ability to swallow secretions
- High risk for altered nutrition: less than body requirements, related to NPO status required by tracheoesophageal fistula and esophageal atresia
- High risk for fluid volume deficit related to NPO status and frequent suctioning
- Anxiety (parental) related to the unknown outcome of surgery

SELECTED REFERENCES

Books

Anderson, K., et al. (Eds.). (1994). *Mosby's medical nursing and allied health dictionary* (4th ed.). St. Louis: Mosby.

Avery, G., and Fletcher, M. (1994). *Neonatology, pathophysiology, and management of the newborn* (4th ed.). Philadelphia, J.B. Lippincott Co.

Bates, B. (1991). *A guide to physical examination* (5th ed.). Philadelphia: J.B. Lippincott Co.

Berkow, R. (ed.). (1992). *The Merck manual of diagnosis and therapy* (16th ed.). Rahway, NJ: Merck Sharp and Dohme Research Laboratories.

Bobak, I. (1992). *Maternity and gynecologic care* (5th ed.). St. Louis: Mosby Year-Book, Inc.

Carpenito, L. (1993). *Handbook of nursing diagnosis* (5th ed.). Philadelphia: J.B. Lippincott Co.

Corbett, J. (1992). *Laboratory tests and diagnostic procedures with nursing diagnosis* (3rd ed.). East Norwalk, CT: Appleton and Lange.

Cunningham, F., et al. (1993). *Williams obstetrics* (19th ed.). East Norwalk, CT: Appleton and Lange.

DeVita, V., et al. (1992). *AIDS—Etiology, diagnosis, treatment, and prevention* (3rd ed.). Philadelphia: J.B. Lippincott Co.

Doenges, M., and Moorhouse, M. (1991). *Nurse's pocket guide: Nursing diagnoses with interventions* (3rd ed.). Philadelphia: F. A. Davis Co.

Gabbe, S., et al. (1991). *Obstetrics: Normal and problem pregnancies* (2nd ed.). New York: Churchill Livingstone.

Gulanick, M., et al. (1994). *Nursing care plans, nursing diagnosis and intervention* (3rd ed.). St. Louis: Mosby.

Iyer, P., Taptich, B., and Bernocchi-Losey, D. (1991). *Nursing process and nursing diagnosis* (2nd ed.). Philadelphia: W.B. Saunders Co.

Jaffe, M., and Melson, K. (1989). *Maternal-infant health care plans.* Springhouse, PA: Springhouse Corp.

Kim, M., et al. (1993). *Pocket guide to nursing diagnoses* (5th ed.). St. Louis: Mosby.

Klaus, M., and Fanaroff, A. (1993). *Care of the high-risk neonate* (4th ed.). Philadelphia: W.B. Saunders Co.

Knuppel, R., and Drukker, J. (1993). *High-risk pregnancy: A team approach* (2nd ed.). Philadelphia: W.B. Saunders Co.

May, K., and Mahlmeister, L. (1990). *Comprehensive maternity nursing: Nursing process and the childbearing family* (2nd ed.). Philadelphia: J.B. Lippincott Co.

Olds, S. (1992). *Maternal newborn nursing* (4th ed.). Redwood City, CA: Addison-Wesley Nursing.

Organization for Ob-Gyn and Neonatal Nurses Staff. (1992). *Core curriculum for maternal-newborn nursing.* S. Mattson and J. Smith (eds.). Philadelphia: W.B. Saunders Co.

Pillitteri, A. (1992). *Maternal and child health nursing: Care of the childbearing and childrearing family.* Philadelphia: J.B. Lippincott Co.

Reeder, S., Martin, L., and Koniak, D. (1992). *Maternity nursing: Family, newborn, and women's health care* (17th ed.). Philadelphia: J.B. Lippincott Co.

Scherwen, L., Scoloveno, M., and Weingarten, C. (1991). *Nursing care of the childbearing family.* Norwalk, CT: Appleton and Lange.

Sparks, S., and Taylor, C. (1993). *Nursing diagnosis reference manual* (2nd ed.). Springhouse, PA: Springhouse Corp.

Thomas, C. (Ed.). (1993). *Taber's cyclopedic medical dictionary* (17th ed.). Philadelphia: F.A. Davis Co.

Whaley, L., and Wong, D. (1994). *Whaley and Wong's nursing care of infants and children* (5th ed.). St. Louis, Mosby Year-Book, Inc.

Wong, D., and Whaley, L. (1990). *Clinical manual of pediatric nursing* (3rd ed.). St. Louis: Mosby Year-Book, Inc.

Periodicals

Bear, K., and Tigges, B. (1993). Management strategies for promoting successful breast-feeding. *The Nurse Practitioner,* 18(6), 50-60.

Campinha-Bacote, J., and Bragg, E. (1993). Chemical assessment in maternity care. *American Journal of Maternal/Child Nursing,* 18(1), 24-28.

Centers for Disease Control. (1993). Update: Barrier protection against HIV infection and other sexually transmitted diseases. *Morbidity and Mortality Weekly Report,* 42(30), 589-600.

Cohn, J. (1993). Human immunodeficiency virus and AIDS: 1993 update. *Journal of Nurse-Midwifery,* 38(2), 65-85.

Cosner, K., and deJong, E. (1993). Physiologic second-stage labor. *American Journal of Maternal/Child Nursing,* 18(1), 38-43.

Curry, L., and Gibson, L. (1992). Congenital hip dislocation: The importance of early detection and comprehensive treatment. *The Nurse Practitioner,* 17(5), 49-55.

DeFerrari, E., et al. (1993). Nurse-midwifery management of women with human immunodeficiency virus disease. *Journal of Nurse-Midwifery,* 38(2), 86-96.

Donaher-Wagner, B., and Braun, D. (1992). Infant cardiopulmonary resuscitation for expectant and new parents. *American Journal of Maternal/Child Nursing,* 17(1), 27-29.

Fleming, B., Munton, M., Clarke, B., and Strauss, S. (1993). Assessing and promoting positive parenting in adolescent mothers. *American Journal of Maternal/Child Nursing,* 18(1), 32-37.

Janke, J. (1993). The incidence, benefits, and variables associated with breast-feeding: Implications for practice. *The Nurse Practitioner,* 18(6), 22-32.

Jay, N. (1993). Gynecologic issues of women with HIV infection. *AWHONN's Clinical Issues in Perinatal and Women's Health Nursing,* 4(2), 258-264.

Ladebauche, P. (1992). Unit-based family-support groups: A reminder. *American Journal of Maternal/Child Nursing,* 17(1), 18-21.

Long, C. (1992). Teaching parents infant CPR—Lecture or audiovisual tape? *American Journal of Maternal/Child Nursing,* 17(1), 30-32.

Meier, P., et al. (1993). Breast-feeding support services in the neonatal intensive-care unit. *Journal of Obstetric, Gynecologic, and Neonatal Nursing,* 22(4), 338-347.

Minkoff, H., and DeHovitz, J. (1991). Care of women infected with the human immunodeficiency virus. *Journal of the American Medical Association,* 266(16), 2253-2258.

Parkman, S. (1992). Helping families say good-bye. *American Journal of Maternal/ Child Nursing,* 17(1), 14-17.

Penny, D., and Perlis, D. (1992). Shoulder dystocia: When to use suprapubic or fundal pressure. *American Journal of Maternal/Child Nursing,* 17(1), 34-36.

Porcher, F. (1992). HIV-infected pregnant women and their infants: Primary health care implications. *The Nurse Practitioner,* 17(11), 46-54.

Reichert, J., Baron, M., and Fawcett, J. (1993). Changes in attitudes toward cesarean birth. *Journal of Obstetric, Gynecologic, and Neonatal Nursing,* 22(2), 159-167.

Ross, T., and Dickason, E. (1992). Nursing alert: Vertical transmission of HIV and HBV. *American Journal of Maternal/Child Nursing,* 17(4), 192-195.

Starn, J., et al. (1993). Can we encourage pregnant substance abusers to seek prenatal care? *American Journal of Maternal/Child Nuring,* 18(3), 148-152.

Sullivan, J., Boudreaux, M., and Keller, P. (1993). Can we help the substance abusing mother and infant? *American Journal of Maternal/ Child Nuring,* 18(3), 153-157.